WHY CHOOSE HOME BIRTH

WHY CHOOSE

CHOOSE

Home Birth

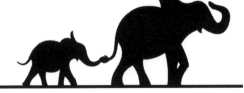

Yes, It's an Option, and Yes, It's Right for Women Today

MONIKA STONE

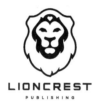

LIONCREST
PUBLISHING

WHY CHOOSE HOME BIRTH

Yes, It's an Option, and Yes, It's Right for Women Today

ISBN   978-1-5445-0353-0 *Hardcover*

978-1-5445-0334-9 *Paperback*

978-1-5445-0335-6 *Ebook*

To my husband, Bill, who sees me and loves me as I am.

To my son, Josef, who made me a mother and changed everything.

To my daughter, Sofia, who journeys with fierceness in her heart and inspires me to be more.

I love each one of you as you are and more than you will ever know.

Contents

Introduction

Are you health conscious, aware of food choices, questioning norms at times, and entering the world of pregnancy and birth? Then this book is for you.

Have you given birth before and felt harmed, hurt, or simply not well supported by the medical system? Then this book is for you.

Have you been informed that your family member is choosing to birth their baby in a home birth setting, and you want to know more? Then this book is for you.

Are you a medical practitioner who has heard about home birth but is not sure what to make of it? Then this book is for you.

Each year in the United States, around four million babies are born. Fifty-five thousand of those babies are born at home into the hands of midwives.

There are two models of care under which we can birth our babies. The one most people utilize is called the medical model of care for childbirth. The lesser-known model is the midwifery model of care for childbirth. You are likely not as familiar with the midwifery model of care.

I am a midwife, and I am inviting you on a journey with me into the world of home birth. This book is written from my personal experience and expertise in accordance to the midwifery model of care, which should be reflective of how home birth midwives practice in states where midwifery is legal.

First, I will debunk the incorrect association of home birth with death and despair. Then I will explain the history of home birth and the history of midwifery. I will explain our credentials. I will give you access to my work as a home birth midwife and explain in detail what prenatal care with a midwife looks like. I will cover the work midwives do during the birthing process and the comprehensive care we provide in the postpartum period.

Most importantly, this book will help you understand the midwifery model of care so that you are able to talk to your family members about it and guide you toward finding the right midwife for you.

I have absolutely no intention to discredit the medical model of care. I am deeply grateful to work in a city where I have access to the medical system and its providers when I need them. This access makes me a better provider and makes home birth safer.

My desire in writing *Why Choose Home Birth* is to open the door to home birth to a greater population. Women and families have choices in childbirth. How can they choose if they do not understand their choices?

Women, babies, and families deserve to have choices in childbirth. The health and well-being of the mother and baby are my number one priority.

The main purpose of this book is to bring awareness to home birth and to normalize home birth as a viable option for women and children. This book will give the reader tools to find a professional, skilled midwife.

Is Home Birth Safe?

Let's address the elephant in the room—the safety of home birth!

I like to address home birth safety with the following statement: "Just because you are choosing a home birth does not mean you are reckless and putting your safety and the baby's safety at risk. Your safety and the baby's safety are my number one concern."

There are numerous quality studies confirming that home birth is a safe birthing option for mom and baby. The fact is, home birth is very safe.

The problem is not safety. The problem is that midwifery and home birth have an image problem.

For many generations, we have been told that home birth is a thing from the past, associated with death and despair, and that a hospital is the safest place to birth a baby. In chapter 1, I discuss the history of hospital birth, which shines a light on the evolution from home birth to hospital birth.

The unspoken truth is that women and babies are harmed in hospital settings as well as out-of-hospital settings. The US has the highest rate of maternal death in the Western civilized world. *These statistics are related to hospital births.* This fact is underreported, yet when out-of-hospital births have negative outcomes, the story is easily picked up by the media.

We have a double standard. It is more likely that you will find negative press on midwives who provided poor care in their out-of-hospital work than on a doctor who provided poor care in a hospital setting. The press leads us to believe that midwives are solely responsible for bad outcomes. The reality is that we have obstetricians who provide poor care with bad outcomes as well.

Pregnancy and birth are two of the most emotionally charged events in one's life. And yes, it's true—women and babies can be harmed and/or die in pregnancy, in childbirth, or postpartum *no matter where the babies are born.* I will absolutely not argue with this reality.

Just as there is bad hospital care, there are also midwives who provide poor care and have bad outcomes. It is important to understand that the midwifery profession is not immune to the reality of unprofessional providers.

So I ask you to please keep an open mind. Midwives are a small group with very little power, attached to a strong image problem, and therefore are an easy target for an emotionally charged article in the Sunday morning paper.

The midwives in my community do their work to make a difference in a woman's life. They serve selflessly and with passion. Midwives don't become midwives to harm and hurt women and babies. Midwives become midwives to listen, respect, love, and provide excellent care to women and babies.

Women who seek midwives are often well-educated, informed, and looking for alternative care. Some have been hurt and/or disillusioned by prior hospital births, and while searching for another way to birth they came across midwifery. There are many reasons women seek midwives.

I wrote this book to shine a light on the midwifery model of care to give you unprecedented insight into my work as a home birth midwife. My hope is that you become informed about your choices in childbirth and that you go on to make an informed decision about the setting and provider that is best for you.

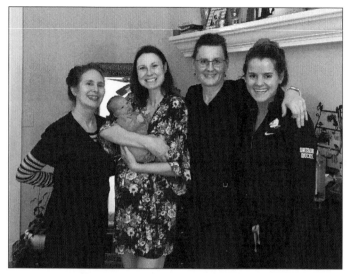

Two hours after giving birth at home, this mom requested to be standing in the picture. She had her first baby via C-section and two vaginal births afterwards.

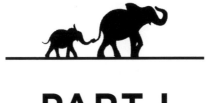

PART I

Know Your Options

///

Chapter 1

///

What a Hospital Birth Looks Like

AMY'S STORY

Amy cries out with relief and joy as the nurse lays her baby boy in her arms.

After twenty-four hours of labor, her birth journey has ended with the big moment of meeting her baby. Her doctor, whom she met only a few minutes earlier, flashes a quick smile and busies himself with delivering the placenta.

Let's have a look at Amy's story from the beginning. She is a healthy mom in her thirties, had no trouble getting pregnant, and was surprised how quickly she became pregnant. She went regularly to her well woman exams and had a doctor she liked. She was happy that she had found someone years ago that she trusted for this pregnancy.

The pregnancy had been great. She ate well, exercised, read all the usual books, and went to birth classes, which were offered through the hospital. Going into the birth, she was not sure if she wanted an epidural or not, but she decided to keep an open mind.

As Amy got closer to her due date, her doctor offered to schedule an induction date for a few days after the due date. Her doctor was on call that day and would see her through the delivery. Amy felt big and tired of the pregnancy, and she liked the thought of being done and having the event scheduled. That took a lot of stress away from worrying about suddenly going into labor.

Amy reported to the hospital on the scheduled night and was told her cervix was only slightly dilated. Another doctor, one she had not met, put her on medication to help ripen her cervix. She was supposed to go to sleep, but the hospital bed felt uncomfortable and she was anxious about the unknown experience that lay ahead. Her husband slept on a bench in the room.

In the morning, the nurse started a Pitocin drip to help start contractions. The medication Amy had received the night before had worked as planned to dilate her cervix and the nurse said the induction should work well. Then the nurse said goodbye and a different day-shift nurse came in.

A few hours after starting the Pitocin, Amy started feeling contractions. She had a monitor on her belly to measure contractions and a monitor to measure baby's heartbeat.

She was wearing a hospital gown, which hung open at the back, exposing her nakedness, and made her feel uncomfortable every time she got out of bed.

When she first arrived, an IV was placed for fluids and some nourishment, as she was not allowed to drink or eat. Due to the IV tubing, the monitors on her belly, and the gaping gown, she decided to not move much and stay in bed.

A few hours after the Pitocin drip started, she felt her first contractions. They were five minutes apart, lasting sixty seconds. Her doctor, who had peeked in for a few minutes in the morning, was happy about the contraction pattern.

Amy decided to get an epidural when she was three centimeters along and had had contractions for about two hours. The contractions came frequently and felt strong. The anesthesiologist came in and worked quickly and was nice. Amy does not even really remember him. She was just happy she got relief from the pain.

As the day went on, she and her husband watched movies and slept. She sucked on some ice chips when her growling tummy was bothering her. She loved her epidural, as she did not feel much. The nurse came every few hours to help her switch positions, empty the catheter, and check her cervix. As the day went on, Amy made steady progress.

By nighttime, she was ready to push. A new night-shift nurse came on. Amy said goodbye to the lovely nurse she had had all day.

The new nurse explained how to push. After a learning curve Amy got the hang of it. The nurse directed her when and how to push, as Amy could not feel her legs nor had any sensation below her belly button.

Her doctor, whom she had known for years, peeked in and said goodbye as her shift was ending. She wished Amy good luck.

After a few hours of steady pushing and very hard work Amy was very close and so ready to be done. The nurse directed her to stop pushing. The bottom part of the bed was broken down. Her legs were re-situated in stirrups. The nurse called everyone to the delivery. Several new faces appeared. One said he was the doctor taking over for her doctor.

Amy did not really care at that moment.

The new doctor gowned up and put all sorts of gear on, washed off Amy's bottom, which was lying at the edge of the broken-down bed. Amy's legs were covered in paper. Everyone got situated in the room. Bright lights were turned on and pointed toward her vagina. Her nurse directed her to push, and after a few good pushes, Amy's baby boy was born. He gave a lusty cry, his cord was cut, and he was placed on Amy's belly.

After the placenta was delivered, the doctor sutured Amy's bottom, flashed a quick smile followed by a congratulations, and was out the door. The bed was being put back together.

The baby was across the room. The nurses checked him out, gave him his newborn medications, and weighed him. He was then bundled up and placed in Amy's arms. She now was a mother. It was such a special moment for her.

MEDICAL-MODEL BIRTH STATISTICS

Per a national statistics report published June 2, 2016,

the number of births for the United States in 2015, was 3,977,745.

In the United States of America, the majority of babies are born in the hospital—around 98 percent. Laboring and giving birth in a hospital is the socially accepted norm for having a baby in the US.

Little girls and boys grow up knowing they were born in a hospital and that is where their siblings were born. The hospital is where they will go to have a baby. Children pick up this understanding while growing up. Giving birth in a hospital is woven into the fabric of our society. With that comes the natural conclusion that having a baby in a hospital is the social norm.

Hospitals are considered the safest place to give birth. They have trained doctors, nurses, and anesthesiologists with every resource available for emergencies, including access to an operating room. The availability of pain medicine via epidurals makes the hospital a great choice for women who desire pain relief in childbirth.

Per recent statistics, a woman who is receiving prenatal care through her ob-gyn has a 23 percent likelihood of labor being induced. This means twenty-three out of every one hundred women will be scheduled for an induction. The reasons cited for induction include no labor around the due date, medical necessity, and patient request.

A pregnant woman walking into a hospital has a 63 percent likelihood of getting an epidural—that's more than half of all pregnant women.

Roughly twelve out of one hundred pregnant women will get an episiotomy, meaning these women will have their perineum cut during birth.

Every third pregnant woman walking into a hospital will have a C-section in the US. The C-section rate has been steady at 32 percent for US women.

WHEN DID WE START GIVING BIRTH IN A HOSPITAL?

Throughout most of history, women attended women giving birth.

The Bible is the earliest document that talks about midwives attending births. Midwives were (and still are) the norm in Europe. They traveled to the New World and attended the births of the early settlers. During colonial times, midwives attended the majority of women delivering babies. These were women who were trained by another midwife and the knowledge and wisdom were passed down from one generation to the next. We do not have full statistics on their outcomes, of course, but all the journals and records midwives kept during those times show around 95 percent success rate for midwife-attended home births.

With the rise of doctors in the late eighteenth century, birth attendance moved from midwives to doctors. With the establishment of medical schools and hospitals, physicians gained credibility. Professional organization through the American Medical Association (AMA) and a campaign for hospital birth and against midwives in home birth changed the landscape in the twentieth century.

In 1900, less than 5 percent of babies were born in the hospital. Over the next century, the medical profession established itself as the professionals of birth. Middle- and upper-class women considered birthing at home something relegated to the lower class. They wanted a pain-free hospital birth.

By 1935, roughly 37 percent of women gave birth in a hospital. Eventually, twilight sleep was introduced and promised a pain-free birth. Medical and hygiene improvements, especially in the field of surgery, established hospitals as safe places to give birth.

In just fifteen short years, the number of hospital births

had more than doubled to 88 percent in 1950, thanks to the introduction of universal medical insurance, which covered hospital births.

Midwives failed to organize and establish midwifery as a respected profession, as it was still in Europe, so as doctors took over, the number of midwives fell dramatically. Rural midwives retired and new midwives did not follow. Immigrant midwives in the first half of the twentieth century, who were professionally trained in European midwifery schools, did continue to attend birth in their own communities, but did not share a common language or attempt to create a national association and midwifery education program. Doctors campaigned against them; calling them "ignorant" and making them look like vestiges of the past that should be left behind in the modern world. This led us to where we stand today—with about 98 percent of women having babies in a hospital setting in the United States.

It was in the 1970s and 1980s that direct-entry midwives founded their first professional organizations, developed educational programs, and created minimum standards of licensure, which subsequently led to a rise in home births.

But what about those 1.36 percent of women having their babies outside of the hospital?

Did they miss the memo?

Are they crazy or reckless?

Or maybe there is another way to give birth?

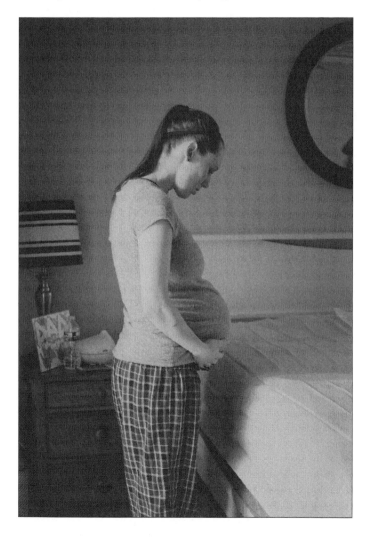

//

Chapter 2

//

Introduction to Home Birth

LISA'S STORY

Lisa is a thirty-year-old woman who is well educated and has a thriving career. She lives with her husband in a beautiful suburban home. They were ready to become parents.

The couple was surprised by how easily Lisa conceived. When she became pregnant with her first child, she started seeing the doctor who had taken care of her over the years. During her first visit, she felt rushed and not as supported as she would have liked to be.

She told a friend about her experience, and that friend recommended she see a midwife. Lisa did not know that she had options when it came to where she gave birth.

When she did research, she discovered several birth centers in town and numerous home birth midwives. Her partner agreed to meet some of them. After touring birth centers and interviewing a handful of home birth midwives, they decided to have a home birth.

Lisa's parents were excited for the home birth after they learned about the process, while her husband's parents were equally anxious about the idea of a home birth.

Lisa loved her hour-long appointments with her midwife, where all her questions were answered. She always left feeling listened to and cared for and therefore felt good about her pregnancy and upcoming birth.

Lisa did, however, remain nervous about the pain of childbirth. She wanted to keep her option for an epidural (and hospital birth) open. Her midwife acknowledged her concern and shared her wisdom of helping many women through the process, but she also reassured Lisa that she would respect her desire to move to the hospital for pain relief if she wanted it.

Lisa went into labor about ten days after her official due date. Her midwife was very calm about her post-date pregnancy and reassured her that this was the norm. Over the first twenty-four hours, Lisa had mild to moderate contractions that were spaced out. The midwife supported her via phone with lots of reassurance and advice. She even stopped by the house to check on Lisa and baby.

Lisa rested, ate, walked, and watched lots of funny movies. Eventually, her contractions got stronger and the midwife came over.

Lisa had to work harder now, as the contractions came closer together and were stronger. She loved walking around, dancing, using the shower, and lying down when she needed a rest. The midwife and her student checked heart tones frequently and took vital signs regularly. They reassured Lisa and her husband.

As contractions got very close and the space in between them was about two minutes, Lisa got into the birth pool. She loved the warm water and floating in it. It instantly helped her better cope with the pain. Lisa felt so many new sensations that she was unable to communicate. She felt like her midwife seemed to know magically what to say. Lisa felt very loved by her husband and her birth team. She was encouraged to listen to her body and do whatever made her most comfortable.

Lisa was also given lots of choices and advice. Someone was always touching and loving on her.

Eventually, a second midwife came over to help with the

birth. When Lisa started pushing, it felt normal and natural to her, as her body just took over.

As the baby was being born, her partner was able to help with the birth, and her baby boy was instantly placed on her chest.

Lisa was so happy to be finished and joyful to meet her son. Her journey took about forty-eight hours.

To Lisa, time had become warped and did not matter. The midwives quietly checked on mom and baby. The placenta was delivered about fifteen minutes after the baby was born and placed in a bag next to mom and baby. The midwives had not yet cut the cord.

One of the midwives checked for perineal tearing. Lisa needed a few stiches in her perineum, but the midwife decided nursing was a priority now and helped get the baby latched. The midwives checked blood pressure, temperature, pulse, and bleeding as Lisa was nursing her baby boy. The midwives listened to the baby's heart rate and lungs frequently, checked temperature as baby was suckling on Mom's breast and snuggling against her.

About forty minutes later, after Lisa had a chance to bond with her baby boy, drink water, and snack, the midwife used lidocaine to numb her perineum and quietly sutured.

Lisa was still holding her baby boy, who had not left her once since he was initially placed on her chest. For the next hour, the couple bonded with their baby.

The midwives quietly cleaned up and were mostly in the other room. When Lisa's son was two hours old, she had eaten a large home-cooked meal, had drunk plenty of fluid, and was ready to get up to go to the bathroom.

The midwives helped her to the bathroom to take a shower. Lisa was surprised how great she felt. While she was bathing, the midwives changed the linens and prepared for the newborn exam.

Lisa returned to her bed, and her baby received his first checkup at the foot of the bed. Lisa and her partner watched the exam and especially loved when he was put in a sling and weighed. He came in at a healthy eight pounds and six ounces.

The midwives continued to clean up and quietly move their bags out. They helped to latch him once more, tucked the couple into bed, and then left quietly.

Lisa reflected that the birth was painful, but she was surprised to realize that it never dawned on her to get an epidural. She felt safe and comfortable at home. She had built a relationship with her midwives and trusted them as her care providers. As she was thinking those thoughts, she slipped into a deep sleep with a heart full of joy and gratitude.

THE MYTH OF THE PAIN-FREE BIRTH BY HEROIC WOMAN

Pain and childbirth are inseparable. They are linked together in our minds and reaffirmed through TV, social media, our own upbringing, and social conversations. Nobody likes to be in pain, so avoiding pain in childbirth seems quite natural for most of us.

Then why do women choose to give birth at home, where the option for pain relief is not available?

Birth is intense and painful. Women birthing at home commit to accepting the sensations they are feeling in their bodies and decide to move through it. They are not especially courageous or heroic. Women giving birth at home are health conscious, proactive in their healthcare needs, like to play an active role during pregnancy, and question norms.

In 2009, when I moved from hospital birth (where I supported women as a doula for eight years) to home birth as a midwife student, I noticed that women at home coped much better with the intensity of birth.

Most people make the assumption that the epidural is the only way to relieve the pain of childbirth. This is a misconception.

Warm water is an analgesic. The safety of a familiar environment with familiar people is an analgesic. Having control over your environment reduces anxiety and promotes relaxation. Think about it—what if you had the ability to turn off lights and have silence or soft music instead of bright lights and abrasive alarms, or the sound of unfamiliar people walking in and out of your room? What if you had a provider you have a relationship with? One that you know and trust versus a complete stranger? The ability to control your environment reduces anxiety, and therefore pain.

As a doula, I observed that women in the hospital had a strong internal struggle about whether to get an epidural or continue with their plan of unmedicated birth.

I always compared the internal struggle to wandering in the desert for days without water, and you're thirsty, very thirsty. Someone comes along and offers you a glass of ice water. Would you decline? Of course not.

All women are concerned about the pain and intensity of childbirth. Home-birthing moms are not different! They wonder if they can handle the pain. They wonder what the pain is like. They remember the pain of prior child-birth. They choose to accept the pain and intensity as part of their birthing experience and how they choose to bring life into the world.

Why are only a little over 1 percent of births happening *out* of hospital?

Safety, meaning a healthy outcome for mom and baby, is the primary concern to women and families giving birth. Over time, home birth has developed a reputation of not being safe, meaning that mother or baby, or possibly both, are getting harmed during the process.

The research (and corresponding data) does not support this concern. Contrary to popular belief, home birth, when attended by *trained, skilled professionals*, is very safe for mother and baby.

It is important to distinguish planned home birth with trained, skilled, professionally licensed midwives from unassisted home birth. In unassisted home birth, the women and families did not receive prenatal care and do not have a licensed midwife present at the birth.

I would like to be clear that I do not endorse unas-sisted home birth. Further, when this book mentions home birth, it is in support of planned home birth with skilled, trained, professionally licensed midwives only.

As stated earlier, the socially accepted way of giving birth is in a hospital setting. Society tends to follow social and cultural norms that are practiced by the majority. The majority of women are not even aware that home birth is an option or that they have a choice in who will care for them prenatally and during childbirth.

Just as society discriminates against the home birth setting, so, too, do insurance companies. Prenatal care by a midwife, home birth, and postpartum follow-up are often not covered by health insurance. Therefore, women who might otherwise choose a home birth but do not have the financial means to pay out of pocket are often left with no choice but to follow the traditional path: an ob-gyn for prenatal care, a hospital birth, and follow-up care by a pediatrician.

Home birth midwives are legal, licensed, and regulated in thirty-two states. In some, they are alegal, meaning that they are not licensed or regulated. In a few states, home birth midwifery practice is illegal, despite the long-term efforts of the midwives in those states to achieve legalization, licensure, and regulation. Over the last decade, more states have legalized home birth midwives. Despite this advancement, there are still only a small percentage of midwives practicing in the US in comparison to ob-gyns. Therefore, access to home birth remains limited.

In 2010, there were 33,624 general ob-gyns in the United States. These providers attended hospital births, with the exception of a very few obstetricians who do attend home births.

According to the American Midwifery Certification Board, in 2017, there were 11,194 certified nurse-midwives (CNMs) and ninety-seven certified midwives (CMs). Around eight thousand CNMs are in practice. The vast majority of these midwives attend hospital births, with only around two hundred CNMs attending out-of-hospital-births.

Per the North American Registry of Midwives (NARM), in 2014, there had been 2,454 Certified Professional Midwife (CPM) certificates awarded. These are primarily the midwives who attend home births or birthing center births.

HOW MIDWIVES ARE EDUCATED AND CREDENTIALED

Midwives have very unique credentialing options, with roots in the history of midwifery across the United States. The Certified Nurse-Midwife and Certified Midwife have their roots in nursing. The Certified Professional Midwife originated from the practice of direct entry midwives.

CERTIFIED PROFESSIONAL MIDWIFE

These are knowledgeable, skilled, and professional primary maternity care providers for women in the child-bearing year.

Certified professional midwives are trained and credentialed to offer expert care, education, counseling and support to women for pregnancy, birth, and the postpartum period. CPMs practice as autonomous health professionals working within a network of relationships with other maternity care providers who can provide consultation and collaboration when needed. All certified professional midwives meet the standards for certification set by the North American Registry of Midwives or NARM (www.narm.org).

The National Commission for Certifying Agencies (NCCA), the accrediting body of the Institute for Credentialing Excellence (ICE, formerly NOCA), accredits the certified professional midwife credential issued by NARM. The mission of ICE is to promote excellence in credentialing for practitioners in all occupations and professions. The NCCA accredits many healthcare credentials, including the certified nurse-midwife (CNM).

The NCCA encourages their accredited certification programs to have an education evaluation process so candidates who have been educated outside of established pathways may have their qualifications evaluated for credentialing. The NARM Portfolio Evaluation Process (PEP) meets this recommendation. The CPM is the only NCCA-accredited midwifery credential that includes a requirement for out-of-hospital experience.

CERTIFIED NURSE-MIDWIFE AND CERTIFIED MIDWIFE

CNMs are educated in two disciplines: midwifery and nursing. They earn graduate degrees, complete a midwifery education program accredited by the Accreditation Commission for Midwifery Education (ACME), and pass a national certification examination administered by the American Midwifery Certification Board (AMCB) to receive the professional designation of CNM. CMs are educated in the discipline of midwifery. They earn graduate degrees, meet health and science education requirements, complete a midwifery education program accredited by ACME, and pass the same national certification examination as CNMs to receive the professional designation of CM.

CNMs and CMs must demonstrate that they meet the Core Competencies for Basic Midwifery Practice of the

American College of Nurse-Midwives (ACNM) upon completion of their midwifery education programs and must practice in accordance with ACNM Standards for the Practice of Midwifery. ACNM competencies and standards are consistent with or exceed the global competencies and standards for the practice of midwifery as defined by the International Confederation of Midwives. To maintain the designation of CNM or CM, midwives must be recertified every five years through AMCB and must meet specific continuing education requirements.[1]

Nurse-midwives often work in doctors' offices and deliver at hospitals or birth centers.

A certified professional midwife CPM is a knowledgeable, skilled, and professional independent midwifery practitioner who has met the standards for certification set by NARM and is qualified to provide the midwifery model of care. The CPM is the only midwifery credential that requires knowledge about and experience in out-of-hospital settings.

Certified professional midwives are not able to work in hospitals or doctors' offices. They tend to work in

1   American College of Nurse-Midwives, *Definition of Midwifery and Scope of Practice of Certified Nurse-Midwives and Certified Midwives*, 2011, http://www.midwife.org/ACNM/ files/ACNMLibraryData/UPLOADFILENAME/000000000266/Definition%20of%20 Midwifery%20and%20Scope%20of%20Practice%20of%20CNMs%20and%20CMs%20 Feb%202012.pdf.

freestanding birth centers or have their own home birth practice.

There are different routes of education for midwives, which lead to very qualified professionals attending births.

HIRING A LICENSED AND SKILLED MIDWIFE

Studies show that home births with a licensed and skilled midwife have good outcomes. There are different pathways to becoming licensed as a midwife. Most home birth midwives are direct-entry midwives and carry the Certified Professional Midwife (CPM) or Licensed Midwife (LM) credential. In hiring a midwife who only became recently certified, check with her if she continues to be mentored and how long she apprenticed. Ask difficult questions, such as "How many births have you attended? What were your outcomes?" More on what questions to ask in chapter 8.

HISTORY OF MIDWIFERY

Women have been the primary support for other women during labor and childbirth for centuries. Women passed on the wisdom of midwifery from one generation to another. The elder midwife had an apprentice whom she passed her knowledge on to. The wisdom around herbal healing, labor, birth, postpartum, and newborn care was passed down from generation to generation. The midwives were regarded as "wise women" at one point, and witches at other points in history.

Midwives are mentioned in the Bible as early as the book of Genesis. They play a significant role in the book of Exodus. In order to keep the Hebrew population down during captivity in Egypt, Pharaoh ordered the midwives Shifrah and Puah to kill all firstborn male children of Hebrew women. The midwives did not execute Pharaoh's order. When Pharaoh asked them why they were not fulfilling his order, the midwives stated that the Hebrew women were strong and the babies had been born before the midwives arrived. This practice led to Moses being saved during this era and subsequently leading his people out of captivity.

As we travel through time, we find great persecution of the midwives in Europe during the Middle Ages from the fourteenth to the seventeenth centuries. Their wisdom around healing, in combination with their female gender, made them mysterious and scary. It gave women knowledge and power, which was threatening in a woman. This often led to witch hunts and many wise women being burned at the stake.

This period results in the suppression of female healers and the rise of the new male medical profession. What started as a clash between men and women had evolved into a war between classes, with midwives serving the peasant population, and the profession of medicine (i.e., early physicians) serving the ruling elite.

As the medical profession developed through the centuries, women were left behind. Doctors trained through universities became the accepted norm. Women were not allowed to train at a university, and therefore midwives became lay practitioners who were hunted, ridiculed, and prosecuted through the centuries.

As the centuries passed and societies changed, the concept of university-trained physicians as the socially accepted healers has remained. At times, midwives were tolerated. At other times, they were persecuted. But they were no longer accepted as healers.

Methods of persecution and discrediting changed with the social norms of the times, but the concept of male-dominated medicine and the disregard for the female midwife remained constant.

Midwives survived the turbulent times in Europe, where they remain the primary attendants at birth in almost all European countries today, and continued to practice as waves of Europeans migrated to the New World. For two centuries, midwives remained commonplace as they guided the first generations of the colonizing Americans into the world.

Europeans weren't the only immigrants to import the art of midwifery to the New World. Slaves arriving from Africa also brought with them long and powerful traditions of midwifery. In African societies, the midwife was typically past childbearing age and worked alongside her teacher—the elder granny midwife.

Black granny midwives played a crucial role in delivering babies in the southern United States. In this era, their persecution was not only for being female, but also for being black. They were almost completely phased out of practice by the 1960s.

As physicians organized themselves with the creation of the American Medical Association (AMA) and, later, the American College of Obstetricians and Gynecologists (ACOG) they campaigned against midwives, and the tradition of midwifery was threatened once more. Midwifery was discredited and the medical profession became the social norm.

Midwives, on the other hand, were neither able to organize themselves and establish themselves as professionals nor were they able to withstand the systematic slander of their profession. When midwives retired, there was no new generation of midwives to carry on their knowledge and traditions.

Mary Breckinridge was instrumental in establishing the nurse-midwifery profession in the US. In 1925, after obtaining her nursing and midwifery training in England, she founded the Frontier Nursing Service in Appalachia, now known as the Frontier Nursing University. Then, in 1939, she founded the Frontier Graduate School of Midwifery. She realized the need for educating nurse-midwives to improve the healthcare of women and families in rural America.

Not until the era of the hippies in the 1960s and 1970s did we see a rise of direct-entry midwives once more. The children born under twilight sleep were looking for a different way to give birth to their children. The release of Ina May Gaskin's book *Spiritual Midwifery* in 1975 led to a new generation of midwives who would practice out-of-hospital.

Midwives today deliver babies in hospitals, birth centers, and at home. They are educated at universities and midwifery schools, or learn via three-year apprenticeships. They are licensed by states across the US. CPMs are credentialed by the North American Registry of Midwives (NARM), a daughter organization of Midwives Alliance of North America (MANA). CNMs and CMs are credentialed by the American Midwifery Certification Board (AMCB)—a daughter organization of the American College of Nurse-Midwives (ACNM). Both NARM and AMCB are federally recognized credentialing bodies.

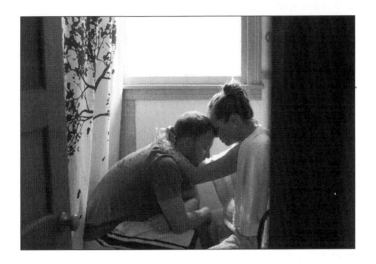

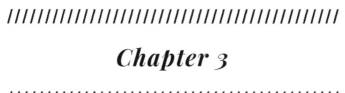

//

Chapter 3

//

Why Home Birth Is Safe

STATISTICS

Home birth has a reputation of being unsafe. Statistics tell a different story.

One of the largest studies presented to date was by the Midwives Alliance of North America (MANA). This study was titled "Outcomes of Care for 16,924 Planned Home Births in the United States: The Midwives of North America Statistics Project, 2004 to 2009."

The results showed that home birth is safe and that the home is a reasonable place to give birth.

Among 16,924 women who planned home births at the

onset of labor, 89.1 percent gave birth at home with a mid-wife. This means these women labored at home and gave birth at home, vaginally and without pain medication.

The intrapartum transfer rate was 10.9 percent. The most common reason for transfer was failure to progress, which means labor was not moving along.

The APGAR scoring system is a standardized method that healthcare professionals use to determine how well baby is transitioning from womb to the outside world. It is an indicator of well-being of baby immediately after birth. In the home births evaluated, APGAR scores taken within the first ten minutes of birth were *ideal* in 98.5 percent of the babies born at home.

Mothers who gave birth at home had a transfer-to-hospital rate after giving birth of just 1.5 percent. The number of babies requiring transfer after birth was even lower, at 0.9 percent.

The majority of babies (86 percent, to be exact) were exclusively breastfeeding at six weeks of age.

My personal practice statistics, which I've tracked since I initially began to practice, closely follow the published data.

I found that 7.3 percent of my clients who started care

with me transferred out prenatally, due to onset of high-risk factors, a change in financial situation, or relocation.

Of the women who labored at home, 85.9 percent successfully delivered at home.

The other 14.1 percent were transferred from home to hospital for non-emergent reasons, primarily prolonged labor.

Out of those clients who started labor at home, 6.1 percent had a C-section. This means my practice has a C-section rate of approximately 6.1 percent.

The rate for preterm labor—as defined by labor starting before thirty-seven weeks' gestation—is 2.7 percent in my practice.

Following birth, the transfer rate for mom is just 0.9 percent and 1.2 percent for baby—all for non-emergent reasons.

When evaluating home birth, it is imperative to look at well-conducted studies as well as a midwife's personal practice statistics to determine if home birth is the right choice for you.

The topic of safety is not as black-and-white as it is often made out to be.

Let's take a journey into the world of midwifery and have a peek behind the curtain, exploring the midwifery model of care for women and families.

Only the healthiest pregnant women get to have a home birth.

Midwives screen mothers who seek a home birth from the moment they cross paths, throughout the pregnancy and during the birth itself.

Chronic illnesses such as high blood pressure, diabetes, genetic illness, and severe obesity are just a few of the conditions that place women at risk for complications during pregnancy and childbirth, and they are therefore not good home birth candidates. Pregnant women who need extended supervision under the medical model of care are better served within that system.

The midwife assesses mother and baby for risk factors on an ongoing basis throughout prenatal care, the birth process, and the postpartum period.

Throughout labor, the midwife continuously monitors the well-being of mother and baby. When variations outside of normal occur, she works on bringing the process back into the range of normal. If labor and birth are not physiological and mother or baby are better served under the medical model of care, the midwife recommends transfer of care into the medical system.

The midwifery model of care uses standardized risk assessment tools and evidence-based protocols for guidance. Ideally, transfer of care to an appropriate provider is recommended when labor is outside the range of normal and long before problems arise.

In order to practice midwifery safely, we need access to the medical model of care. Transferring to a hospital should be a seamless and smooth process for everyone involved in the birthing process.

RISK ASSESSMENT

Risk assessment is a tool utilized by midwives to aid them in recognizing when pregnancy or birth changes from low risk to non-absolute risk or to absolute risk for home birth. This tool assigns various conditions to different risk categories—absolute risk, in which the risk is too high to safely attempt a home birth, and non-absolute risk, which requires consultation with another provider (such as a maternal-fetal medicine physician) but does not necessarily rule out home birth.

In my personal practice, I incorporate standardized risk

assessment tools along with experience, consultation with other midwives, and intuition.

If I have an atypical pregnancy or labor that is still within the range of normal, we move forward. However, if I look at the greater picture and see several issues that, while acceptable individually, can lead to an increased risk for problems when combined, I may recommend transfer of care.

MICHELLE'S STORY

Let's look at Michelle's story. She had a normal birth at home with her first son. Her second pregnancy was uneventful. Michelle was well educated and easy to work with. Her husband was very supportive of the home birth.

Toward the end of her pregnancy, her son's heart rate was consistently in the lower range of normal. She was five days post-date (i.e., past her due date) when labor signs started.

She spent the next three nights and days starting and stopping labor. I checked on her by phone on the first evening, and everything was normal. We expected her to start a strong labor pattern and deliver within the next twelve hours. This did not happen.

During the third night, her contractions were regular

and strong for several hours and then went away. When I checked in with her in the morning, I heard a slight anxiety in her voice, which was unlike her, and noticed a sense of relief when I told her I would be visiting her at home later that day.

When I arrived at Michelle's house, the baby's heart tones were just ten beats below the range of normal. Baby started moving and the heart rate jumped up into the normal range but quickly dropped again. The parents were used to hearing their son for months now and noticed the slower heart rate.

I took a deep breath and started a difficult conversation. First, I recounted how the baby's heart rate in the office for the last two weeks had been on the lower end of normal. Second, we discussed how Michelle was not quite tipping over into labor. Lastly, I pointed out that the baby's heart rate had dropped even lower that day— below the range of what is considered normal. I reassured them that their son was well but recommended we go to the hospital to check on him given the events as a whole. The parents agreed with my recommendation.

It turned out that the placenta was not nourishing the baby boy optimally. Therefore, an induction in the hospital was warranted, and two hours later, a healthy boy was born. The parents were deeply grateful to me for being cautious and taking the time to visit them on a Saturday to ensure the safety of their child.

Transfer of Care Plan for Birth

My range for travel to a home birth is up to a one-hour drive. I serve clientele in urban, suburban, and rural areas. At thirty-six weeks' gestation, I make a visit to the home and create a "transfer of care plan" should the need for a hospital transfer arise. The parents are well informed about the plan.

The plan varies based on where the client lives, but generally speaking, hospitals are chosen that are supportive of midwife transfers. Midwives work very hard to build relationships with hospitals to promote smooth transfers for their clientele. However, the level of support in a hospital setting can vary greatly from state to state. In Texas, where I live, we even see a large variance from county to county.

For urban births, the hospital is often close—about a ten- to fifteen-minute drive. For suburban areas, the hospital may be twenty to twenty-five minutes away. For rural areas, we are often a thirty-minute or more drive away; thus, I've been known to scan for spots to land a helicopter as I navigate the country roads. My students find this humorous, but it's a great lesson in the importance of being prepared for an emergency!

Should the need for a transfer arise, we call 911 for emergent transfers and go by private car for non-emergent transfers. In ten years as a home birth midwife, I have called 911 five times. Each time, it was the smart way to transfer for proper supervision, but neither mom nor baby was in a life-threatening situation.

AMANDA'S STORY

Amanda's story reflects the majority of transfer of care situations that home birth midwives deal with.

Amanda was a healthy first-time mom. Her labor started on the evening of the fifth day past her due date. She rested as much as possible through the night but only dozed off a few times as she was very excited about meeting her baby girl. By morning, her contractions were still about ten minutes apart.

The midwife examined Amanda and discovered she was dilated two centimeters, which was a change from the most recent exam at the office. The midwife encouraged Amanda to eat, drink, walk, nap, and watch funny movies while labor progressed. Toward the evening, contractions were getting closer together and stronger. Amanda found herself breathing and moaning during contractions and resting in between.

The midwife stopped by Amanda's house and found her cervix had progressed to five centimeters, which was a huge change from the morning. The midwife was settling in for the night and began preparing for the birth. Heart tones were checked every thirty minutes; blood pressure, temperature, and pulse were taken every four hours. The team supported Amanda through contractions, encouraged her to move, rest, and utilize water for relaxation and pain relief.

By midnight, Amanda's cervix had opened to seven centimeters (out of the necessary ten centimeters before it would be time to push). The baby was still positioned high in the pelvis. While the midwife could feel that Amanda's baby was head down, she also knew the baby was not perfectly positioned to navigate the pelvis. The midwife recommended positions to encourage the baby to rotate, in addition to homeopathic remedies.

Toward early morning, Amanda appeared tired and the midwife suggested she sleep between contractions. Amanda fell asleep and the contractions started spacing out, which gave her the opportunity to rest. After two hours, Amanda felt much better, requested breakfast, and was ready to keep going.

Upon examination, the midwife discovered that Amanda's cervix had not really changed since midnight, but the baby's head was lower—an encouraging sign.

The midwife discussed the findings with Amanda and her partner, and offered the options of a hospital transfer for pain relief or continuing at home for a few more hours. She also provided reassurance that the baby was doing well but educated the couple that prolonged labor is stressful for both mom and baby.

The midwife prepared the couple for the possibility of a hospital transfer, shifting the frame from the dream of a home birth to a successful vaginal birth with the help of an epidural and Pitocin in the hospital. The parents were given some time to think about their choices and decided to stay home longer.

Amanda spent the next few hours walking, changing positions frequently, and drinking ample fluids and electrolyte drinks. Her contractions returned and she worked through them well. Four hours later, her contractions became strong and Amanda reported lots of pelvic pressure. The midwife checked and found no change in the cervix from the prior exam.

The parents knew it was time to move to the hospital for help. Amanda was exhausted. She had tried having her baby girl at home with courage and strength. Amanda found herself crying a few quiet tears.

Her midwifery team helped her and her partner get ready

to go. Everyone moved about with a quiet purpose. The midwife called the nearby hospital and talked to the charge nurse at the labor and delivery unit. Amanda's records were faxed ahead. When everything was settled, Amanda's partner drove her to the hospital with the midwife following behind. They walked directly to the labor and delivery unit. Amanda was checked in. Within an hour, an epidural was placed, and Amanda loved the pain relief. She found herself sleeping and waiting with her midwifery team and partner at her side.

Finally, at sunset once more, she pushed for an hour and was rewarded by meeting her baby girl. Amanda was overjoyed to finally hold her miracle baby. After the birth, she stayed in the hospital for a few days. When she returned home, the midwife stopped by for a home visit and continued to care for Amanda and baby.

Amanda continues to mourn the loss of her dream of a home birth. Despite this, she is happy with the outcome and grateful she was able to labor at home and receive the support of her midwifery team in the hospital. Amanda loved the prenatal and postpartum care she received from her midwife.

This is a story that most home birth midwives know very well. A first-time mom attempting a home birth, and after a long trial of labor, transferring to the hospital for help. Statistically, these make up the majority of hospital transfers from midwife-led births. The transfer of care is by private car and is non-dramatic. There are no sirens. There is no life-or-death situation. *The outcomes are good.*

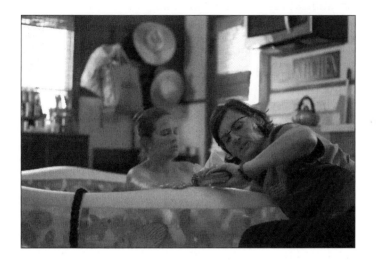

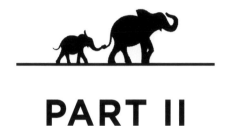

PART II

The Home Birth Experience

Chapter 4

The Midwifery Model of Care

DEFINITION OF THE MIDWIFERY MODEL OF CARE

In the midwifery model of care, the woman is the center of care.

The midwifery model of care is based on the fact that pregnancy and birth are normal life processes.

The Midwives Model of Care is based on the following tenets:

- Monitoring the physical, psychological, and social well-being of the mother throughout the childbearing cycle

- Providing the mother with individualized education, counseling, and prenatal care, continuous hands-on assistance during labor and delivery, and postpartum support
- Minimizing technological interventions
- Identifying and referring women who require obstetrical attention

The application of this woman-centered model of care has been proven to reduce the incidence of birth injury, trauma, and cesarean section.[2]

The midwifery model of care is based on screening women on an ongoing basis for home birth. It all starts with prenatal care.

One of the questions I get frequently is "Are you doing any testing?" I always smile and state, "You are not giving up access to all available testing and treatment just because you are choosing to work with a home birth midwife."

Midwifery clients have access to all testing and treatment available for pregnancy. The difference is that they give informed consent about testing and treatment.

---

2   Midwifery Task Force, "Midwives Model of Care definition," 1996, http://cfmidwifery.org/ mmoc/define.aspx.

PILLARS OF MIDWIFERY-LED CARE

RELATIONSHIP

The midwife and the client are in a partnership role where each has rights and responsibilities in the relationship. Care is provided within the framework of an open dialogue. The midwife explains recommendations for testing and treatment, and shares her protocols for care. The woman is encouraged to research and learn about pregnancy, birth, and the postpartum period. She has a right to question testing and treatment. The midwife explains options for testing and treatment within her scope of practice.

NUTRITION

Nutrition is vital in growing a healthy baby who can tolerate labor. Eating organic whole foods that are prepared at home is vital to nourishing both mother and baby. Nutrition counseling is based on individual dietary preferences. The strategy is to meet the patient where they are at any given period in time. On occasion, we spend an entire pregnancy weaning off soda and junk food, and consider this a success. However, the vast majority of midwifery clients are already very healthy in their food choices and only need a little extra support for the pregnancy.

EXERCISE

Exercise reduces stress, builds stamina for labor and birth, and helps with fetal positioning. Everyone is too busy for exercise; yet, second to nutrition, this is the one thing a pregnant woman can do to increase her chance of an uneventful birth.

MENTAL HEALTH

Midwives spend a lot of time listening to women about their emotions and feelings around pregnancy, parenting, life experiences, and significant relationships. Everyone wants to be heard. Midwives listen.

FACILITATION AND EDUCATION

The midwife is an expert in normal pregnancy and birth, and helps the client plan her individual pregnancy, birth, and postpartum. The midwife helps, guides, and navigates through emotions, sensations, and body changes experienced during pregnancy. The midwife helps prepare the client for birth, breastfeeding, baby wearing, baby sleeping, baby care, and so on.

MARIE'S STORY

Marie had given birth at home three times—all beautiful boys. I helped her with all of her prenatal care, births, and postpartum care. Each pregnancy, birth, and postpartum was different.

Her first pregnancy was normal for a first-time mom. She had lots of questions. The birth was typical—a long early stage of labor followed by a beautiful birth.

It was nice to see the family grow and to take care of them for the second baby. They were seasoned parents and had settled into life with a child. First-time mom questions were replaced by questions about processing life as a family. Her second birth was a water birth. The baby came very fast. When I checked on the baby on the first day after birth, he was breathing too fast but otherwise doing well. The family had to make a trip to the hospital for evaluation. They were able to go home after a few days.

By the third pregnancy, Marie came mostly alone. Her husband was busy working, and her mom helped take care of the boys. Marie enjoyed her alone time with the midwife. The third boy came so quickly that Marie didn't even realize she was in labor. When I arrived at her house, she was busy getting her other boys ready for baseball. I gently directed her to go upstairs and let me evaluate her. The baby was born forty-five minutes later.

Each of Marie's pregnancies was different. Her needs were different. She went through lots of personal growth with each pregnancy. Having cared for Marie through many years and changes, I was able to tailor her care for each individual pregnancy and birth. Being a family midwife is my greatest reward and compliment.

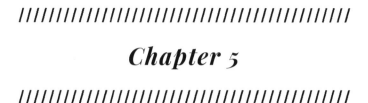

Chapter 5

Prenatal Care with a Midwife

AMY'S PRENATAL CARE

Remember Amy, who gave birth in the hospital? Let's look at her prenatal care under the medical model of care.

As soon as Amy found out she was pregnant, Amy contacted her ob-gyn, who had been her provider for many years. Her initial visit was scheduled soon thereafter.

At the first visit, the receptionist checked Amy in and asked her to take a seat in the waiting room, where she sat for an hour before her name was finally called. An assistant escorted Amy to a busy hallway, where her weight was taken and the number announced aloud for everyone to hear. Next, the assistant showed her to a small, sterile room with an exam table situated starkly in the middle. Amy settled on a piece of paper covering the table. The assistant took her vital signs, asked a few questions, and handed her a gown with directions to undress. This took about five minutes.

Amy undressed and settled back on the paper covering of the table. After thirty minutes, the doctor appeared, smiling at her, and congratulating her on the pregnancy. Then the doctor busied herself doing a sonogram. Amy was able to see the heartbeat. She was very emotional at the reality check of her pregnancy. After the sonogram, her doctor did a pelvic exam. Her doctor congratulated her once more and left the room. After another twenty-minute wait, an assistant walked in and drew Amy's blood. Eventually, someone else came in to instruct Amy about pregnancy precautions, gave her some materials, and told her to get dressed. She went through the front desk to schedule her next appointment and settled her co-pay.

She was seen by her ob-gyn every four weeks until twenty-eight weeks of pregnancy. The visits were quick. Amy made sure that she had her questions written down at each visit so she would not forget them during the short five to ten minutes with her doctor. At twenty-eight weeks, the appointment frequency increased to every other week. By thirty-six weeks of pregnancy, she was asked to undress once more, and her doctor checked her cervix. She was seen weekly from then on, and her cervix was checked at each visit.

At times, she would come to her visit and be informed that she was due for a blood draw or other testing. Some tests were done in the office and some tests were done at the lab. She never heard back about results, so she assumed all was normal.

As Amy approached her due date, she was offered an induction for the day her doctor was on call. She was ready to meet her baby boy and wanted a familiar face during labor, so she scheduled the induction as recommended.

CONTINUOUS CONTINUITY OF CARE

In the midwifery model of care, continuous continuity of care is essential. The term "continuous continuity" explains the concept—the midwife initiates care, provides all prenatal care, attends the birth, and cares for mother and baby after delivery. In summary, the midwife, or a small group practice of midwives, takes care of all aspects of the pregnancy through birth and postpartum. This model allows for a relationship to be formed between the midwife and the client. The use of the term "client" instead of "patient" is intentional. We do not call our clients patients because we do not believe that pregnancy is an illness, and therefore the mother is not a patient.

The relationship that is established between the midwife practice and her client during the continuous continuity of care model is a pillar of the midwifery model of care.

The client is an active participant in care. She manages her nutrition and exercise goals and works on reducing stress in her daily life. The pregnant mom is encouraged to learn about testing and treatment recommended in pregnancy, birth, and postpartum. All testing and treatment is discussed before the recommended time of testing and treatment. The client and her partner are given choices about their care.

I find the majority of my clientele is well educated on recommended testing and treatment and opt to proceed with the standard of care similar to the medical model of care. They feel empowered that procedures are explained in advance and that there is an open dialogue about the risks and benefits of testing—all of which leads to an informed decision about care. If a client decides against certain testing and treatment, they can opt out by signing a waiver. They have done so via an informed decision.

On average, prenatal appointments are one hour long. We check vital signs, weight, and urine. We listen to the baby's heart tones and measure the fundal height (i.e. height of the uterus). Midwives monitor growth and well-being of baby and mom very carefully; however, this is only a fraction of the time spent with the client.

The majority of the appointment is spent talking with the expectant mother, answering questions, providing support, and creating a supportive relationship. Moms like to talk about their pregnancies, children, husbands, and family affairs. They like to be heard and to process ongoing issues that occupy their mind. We also cover nutrition, weight gain expectations, testing and treatment, preparing for birth, and the postpartum period. Each prenatal visit is tailored toward the client's individual need at this particular stage in her pregnancy and life.

Pregnancy is often portrayed as a state of bliss and joy in the media. Pregnant women do experience joyful and blissful pregnancies. But they also deal with anxiety, angst, and fear of the unknown. Their changing bodies come with an influx of hormones and new ailments to adjust to.

In the continuous continuity of care model, the relationship between client and midwife is the cornerstone. The midwife gets to know the mom, and the mom, in turn, gets to know the midwife. Each visit, we're able to pick up where we left off. We continue to work to address mom's social and emotional needs throughout the pregnancy, birth, and postpartum experience.

Prenatal care is designed to evaluate the well-being of mother and baby. When findings are abnormal, the provider formulates a plan of care to return to the range of normal.

In the midwifery model of care, we use lifestyle modifications, homeopathic remedies, herbal tinctures, and teas to heal. Midwives refer to related professionals if the need for additional care arises. We work with endocrinologists, psychologists, perinatal specialists, chiropractors, acupuncturists, and other related professionals to provide co-care for our clients.

I always say, "I know what I know, and I know what I do not know." I am an expert in normal and healthy pregnancy. I am trained and experienced to recognize variations within the range of normal and will provide a care plan to return to that range. When we are unable to return to a normal range with midwifery care or help from related professionals, we refer the client to a physician to continue care and plan a hospital delivery.

SERVICES MIDWIVES PROVIDE

- Comprehensive health history

- Physical exam with Pap smear
- Lab draws and testing
- Monitoring fetal growth and heart tones
- Monitoring the mother with vital signs, urine check, and weight gain
- Routine testing and treatment for pregnancy
- Education for pregnancy, birth, postpartum, baby care, parenting
- Preparation for birth
- Addressing social and emotional complaints like depression and anxiety
- Counseling for nutrition, exercise, stress reduction
- Health and wellness counseling
- Referral for sonograms, diabetes, thyroid care
- Managing expectations and formulating a plan for postpartum care

Prenatal care with a midwife goes far beyond a quick checkup. We build a relationship while supervising a pregnancy. Once the due date arrives, the mother knows her birth team and, having established a trusted relationship, she feels safe with her midwife.

LISA'S PRENATAL CARE

Let's visit with Lisa to discover what her prenatal care looked like under the midwifery model of care.

When Lisa found out she was pregnant, she started care with her ob-gyn but learned through a friend about the midwifery model of care. She eventually opted for a home birth under the care of midwives. Lisa researched online and contacted several local midwives and a birth center whose web presence she liked. After meeting three home birth midwives and touring a birth center, she found the perfect fit. She was excited about her first appointment.

At the day and time of her appointment, Lisa's midwife greeted her in the small and cozy waiting room shortly after arrival. Her midwife offered tea and water as she invited Lisa to sit down in a cozy chair in the middle of her office. They talked about how Lisa had been feeling and reviewed her health history. Next, the midwife checked Lisa's vital signs, listened to the baby's heart tones, and drew blood. The visit lasted about two hours. Lisa left with lots of valuable information about her pregnancy, but with the sound of her baby's heart tones at the top of her mind.

Two weeks later, Lisa returned to the office, where the midwife reviewed her lab results and explained them in detail. Lisa also needed a physical exam. She was able to wear her own shirt and liked that the midwife used sheets instead of paper to cover the exam table. The midwife explained every aspect of the physical exam. She also explained in detail why and how each test was performed. This visit lasted an hour.

Lisa continued to see her midwife every four weeks until twenty-eight weeks of pregnancy, and every two weeks thereafter. At thirty-six weeks, she was seen at home. After the home visit, Lisa was seen in clinic every week.

Her visits usually lasted an hour. They started with a conversation about how she was feeling. Lisa and the midwife discussed nutrition, exercise, and stress management. The midwife always had remedies for common pregnancy ailments, offered an ear for life's challenges, and helped prepare Lisa for the home birth.

Afterwards, the midwife checked Lisa's vitals and listened to the baby's heart tones. Visits always included information about upcoming testing, so Lisa felt well prepared when any tests were performed. She felt empowered to have a voice in her care and the ability to make informed decisions about testing.

Lisa was informed about genetic testing early in her pregnancy and decided to decline testing. At twenty weeks of pregnancy, she had her first and only ultrasound. She enjoyed seeing the baby and was excited to share the images she took home.

The rest of the pregnancy was uneventful. Lisa's due date came and went. She was not worried. Her midwife had often said that most babies come after the due date. Sure enough, Lisa's contractions started one week after Lisa's official due date.

//

Chapter 6

//

Birthing Your Baby at Home with a Midwife

NATURAL AND PHYSIOLOGIC CHILDBIRTH

Witnessing childbirth that unfolds without intervention is a great privilege. The woman's body—which knows how to grow a human infant—also knows how to birth the baby. As a home birth midwife, I trust in a woman's innate ability to birth her baby. I witness beauty, strength, and courage as women move through labor. I see great transformation as they push their babies toward the light. For a moment, all layers grown to protect oneself within society fall away and the true self shines. Birth is raw and honest.

As we leave our homes, we layer up with different behaviors to serve us in different ways. We act one way in a professional setting, another way in a public setting, and yet another way around family. Home is hopefully a place where these layers come off. Where we are the closest to our true self.

If a woman chooses home birth and commits to the process, then this is the environment where the birth hormones unfold best. Interventions become unnecessary. The contractions are strong, and birth follows its natural rhythm. Babies are simply born. I have witnessed this in hundreds of births over ten years.

DUE MONTH

Depending on a midwife's credentials and the individual state of practice, there is generally a window from thirty-seven weeks' gestation to forty-two weeks' gestation in which we can deliver at home. If labor commences before or after this five-week window, women are transferred to a medical provider for a hospital delivery.

It all starts with a due month, rather than a due date. Only about 4 percent of babies are born on their actual due date. Midwives have long been comfortable with a "wait and see" approach. Depending on individual practice guidelines, protocols, and state licensing rules and regulations, midwives tend to wait for babies up to two weeks after the initial due date. This means a baby is considered "due" at forty-two weeks' gestation, not forty weeks.

In my practice, over 95 percent of women see the due date come and go. Few of my clients deliver before their due date. I feel it is a great gift to not rush the birth of the baby, but instead let the baby come on his or her own terms. By 41.5 weeks, most of my clients have given birth.

The physiologic process of what starts labor is not fully understood. In the midwifery model of care, we believe that babies will be born when mom and baby are ready for the next step. Every day of maturation and growth in utero is important for baby. Mom may be very tired of being pregnant and dealing with various ailments. In the midwifery model of care, we discuss the importance of the due month and the great possibility of a post-due-date birth early in pregnancy. We prepare the client throughout the pregnancy to be patient near the end.

Let's pull the curtain back once more and explore what a home birth looks like. Come to a birth with me!

HOW TO GET READY FOR A HOME BIRTH

Preparing for a home birth is simple. We direct clients to prepare bags with the following birth essentials:

- Baby blankets and baby clothes
- Towels and washcloths
- Sheets, two sets
- Postpartum essentials such as wipes, alcohol, cotton pads, diapers, Advil, Tylenol, sitz bath herbs.

Clients are also instructed to order a birth kit that has been curated by the midwife from a medical supplier. The birth kit has all of the disposable items necessary for the birth.

The average home birth produces two loads of laundry and one tall bag of trash. The midwifery team washes the laundry and disposes of the trash before leaving. It's always our goal to leave the house the way we found it, with exception of a baby in mom's arms!

Contrary to popular belief, we have a system in place that prevents ruined mattresses or linens. Home birth is not only safe but also very economical.

UNLIMITED PHONE SUPPORT DURING EARLY LABOR

Midwives understand the importance in recognizing the differences between latent early and active labor. Early labor is a time when contractions are very tolerable for mom—she can walk and talk through them. Yet the contractions are there and it appears they are staying. This stage might last anywhere from a few hours (for moms who have given birth before) to one to three days for first-time moms.

This is often a time of confusion—no matter how many times a woman has given birth. Questions arise, such as "How long will these phases last?" "Do I have enough energy?" and "What will my birth look like?" Moms need guidance and reassurance, and a plan for nutrition, hydration, rest, and activity in place.

Midwives are amazing in supporting moms during early labor. Women have direct access to the midwife via phone. I tend to create a care plan for the whole family from one phone call to the next. The calls are spaced anywhere from fifteen minutes to four hours apart. I educate my clients to call me early and often, so that I can provide guidance and support to set her up for the birth she desires. As a midwife, this helps me plan and guard my energy for the next stage.

THE MIDWIFE COMES TO THE HOME IN ACTIVE LABOR

When contractions become stronger and closer together, it is time for the midwife to be present at the birth. Mom needs the support and the baby's heart tones need to be carefully monitored. My car is always packed and ready to go. Interesting side note: I have not loaded groceries into my trunk in many years.

As I drive to the birth, I think about the family, their desires for this birth, and how their last birth(s) went.

The first few moments after arriving are usually very telling. If mom is comfortably walking around and greets me at the door, it may be early. However, I've also learned that a first impression can be misleading.

I've had moms open the door with big smiles and comfortably walking around at eight centimeters dilation. At the other end of the spectrum, I've found moms in their bedroom appearing as if they are about to give birth who are only two centimeters dilated.

After arrival, when hugs and smiles are exchanged, I listen to baby's heart tones to see how baby is doing. Next, we chat. When everyone is somewhat settled, I check mom's dilation. Based on those findings, a care plan is communicated with the parents. Sometimes labor is early and mom needs a little help learning how to cope with contractions. It is not unusual to make a few trips to check on a first-time mom for extra support.

When a client has a history of a rapid birth, we are vigilant in coming early. I have spent hours with moms in early labor, and within a short time period the contractions changed and the baby was born shortly thereafter. I might not have made it had I not already been there. This is our commitment as midwives to "be with women."

Generally speaking, as midwives we stay with a client when labor is active, which by definition means "accelerated cervical dilation typically beginning at six centimeters" (American College of Obstetrics Guidelines). Early, latent labor (before 6 cm) can safely take one to three days and the midwife will check on mom and baby and offer encouragement and support. However, it's not as black-and-white as "before six centimeters I leave; after six centimeters I stay." This is where a midwife's experience comes into play and is critical in determining when to stay and when to go.

A second-time mom may only be a few centimeters dilated, but her contractions are strong and frequent. In these cases, I tend to settle in. Most of the time, baby comes sooner rather than later. A good understanding of the client's personality, her history, and her desires are all contributing factors in the decision to stay or go.

We always stay if active labor is present. Active labor necessitates *intermittent monitoring*. This is the standard of care recommended by the American College of Obstetrics for low-risk births. It includes an initial set of vital signs on mom and fetal heart tones via a hand-held Doppler for a minimum of ninety seconds every thirty minutes.

We tend to set up for births in the bedroom. The disposable birth kit is opened and sorted, and material is laid out on the dresser in the bedroom. Equipment for vital signs is laid out on the mother's side of the nightstand. The bed is covered with plastic to protect the mattress. Fresh sheets are laid on top of the protected mattress. Another layer of plastic is laid on top of the fresh sheets, and then a final set of sheets is draped over the plastic. The top sheets are the birth sheets. The bottom sheets are the ones mom will recover on.

The "rescue bag" is set up, oxygen is turned on, and equipment is checked.

We place a heating pad into a co-sleeper, baby bassinet, or crib—whichever parents have in the room. The changing table works as well. The heating pad is covered with baby blankets, baby hats, and towels.

The delivery tray holds instruments to clamp and cut—cord clamp, sterile gloves, olive oil, different suction equipment, flashlight, and wipes.

Herbs, homeopathic remedies, and medications are set aside in case they are needed.

The entire setup is portable, and we follow mom wherever it appears she may deliver.

Once all of the equipment is out and ready to go, we listen to baby's heart tones once more and check in with the parents on their desires or needs. We encourage the laboring woman and remind her to hydrate and eat if she desires.

She can labor anywhere she wants to. She can be in any position that feels comfortable. It is up to the laboring woman to choose to be active or rest. At this point, her birth team is invited to the home. This team may include a birth photographer, doula, friend, and/or family members.

Often, the couple desires to labor alone in their bedroom. Sometimes a large group is present. At times, the mom wants her children present. The midwife helps facilitate whatever the mom desires. Prior to the birth, we have talked at length about whom mom wants present and have discussed how to prep everyone.

It is now time for the midwife to start charting. I use electronic health records. It is important to keep excellent records for many reasons, but to name just a few, they help mom process the birth, document my work, and ensure insurance reimbursement. Just like any other healthcare profession, we spend a decent amount of time on documentation.

At this point, about one hour has passed. We settle in for the labor and birth. My birth team has been updated and is ready to come when we get closer to birth. Depending on travel time, mom's progress, and who is assisting me, the birth assistant may already be on her way. When I have a student working with me, she will always come along with me.

LABOR SUPPORT

Time becomes warped during birth. Hours can easily pass by. Patience is a trait any midwife needs to possess and cultivate. I consider it a fast birth and recovery when I stay eight hours at someone's house. It is not uncommon for us to be with our clients twelve to twenty-four hours or longer.

The hours are spent laboring with the mom and partner, giving support and encouragement. We labor with women.

PHYSICAL SUPPORT

The midwife encourages the mom to change positions frequently and offers ideas for positioning. This is helpful for comfort and labor progression. We offer hands-on comfort measures like comforting touch, counterpressure, acupressure, and breathing techniques for the laboring mom. A midwife's skilled hands and positioning tools such as a rebozo (shawl used for helping baby shift into a better position) or a peanut (ball shaped like a peanut) can help with baby's rotation through the birth canal.

EMOTIONAL SUPPORT

During birth, midwives support the entire family, working through the many emotions that arise during labor. I like to help create a space where the hormones of labor can flow easily. Laboring women and their partners will receive encouragement, nurturing, and connection at this tender, vulnerable time in their lives.

PARTNER SUPPORT

Partners need support as well. We make sure the partner has a chance to take care of him/herself. Questions are answered. I find great joy in teaching the partner how to support the laboring mom. My hope is that the partners connect to each other and bond through this experience.

We are conscious of giving the laboring mom and her partner privacy to be together during this special time.

The midwives often stay in the living room. I tend to pass time by doing paperwork or resting; some midwives like to knit. Students typically study.

VAGINAL EXAMS

Vaginal exams give us a lot of insight about how labor progresses, but they are not our only tool. The initial exam is important to give the midwife an idea of mom's starting point. From there, we develop a plan for the birth and when to call the assistant to the birth. In my practice, I try to delay additional vaginal exams for at least four to six hours. In the interim, I'm able to gain insight into mom's progress by monitoring her behavior and contraction pattern.

Let me give you an example. If I have a repeat client with a history of an uneventful first birth in active labor, I primarily rely on her behavior and contraction pattern to assess labor progress. The contractions get stronger as the hours go by; she reports lots of pelvic pressure and eventually gets a strong urge to push. As her midwife, I encourage her to listen to her body and follow its cues, and the baby will be in mom's arms soon. She had only one vaginal exam. Women dislike vaginal exams. In my midwifery practice, I feel a strong obligation to do them as little as possible.

Interestingly, moms often start pushing on their own

when dilation is complete and they are mentally ready for the next stage of birth. At times, moms get a break in contractions and take a nap that gives them the extra energy they need for pushing.

The equipment we bring allows us to care for the labor, birth, and postpartum with safety for mom and baby in mind. It allows us to manage emergencies in a similar manner as they would be managed in the hospital or to stabilize and transfer care to a hospital.

HYDROTHERAPY AKA WATER BIRTH

To my surprise, I recently came across a statement asserting that home birth and water birth were one and the same. While it is true that as a home birth midwife, I consider water a great benefit to my clients (as immersion in a birth pool can aid in pain relief), not all clients choose water birth, and even some who do choose to get out of the water and give birth outside the birth pool.

The dictionary defines water birth as "a birth in which the mother spends the final stages of labor in a birthing pool, with delivery taking place either in or out of the water."

At times my prospective clients ask, "Do I have to have a water birth if I choose a home birth?" The answer is simply "No."

Now that I have cleared up this misunderstanding, let's look at the benefits of utilizing water in labor during a home birth. Water:

- Offers significant pain relief and promotes relaxation.
- Promotes mobility and frequent position changes.
- Helps labor progress more quickly.
- Laboring women enjoy the birth pool as a protected space.

These benefits, which I have come to know in my ten years of facilitating water births, are yet another significant reason to choose an out-of-hospital birth.

In my practice, I offer a birth pool to all my clients in an effort to promote water birth. We discuss how to set up the pool for water birth, when to utilize the pool, and how to set realistic expectations.

Planning for a Water Birth

The birth pools themselves are designed to be deep for buoyancy, are sturdy enough to hold the water, are easy to set up and take down, and are made to be sanitized. For home birth, we need to utilize these pools instead of tubs, as tubs do not give the full benefit of water birth. Tubs can give the benefit of warm water but not the buoyancy and freedom of movement. During my home visit at thirty-six weeks, I help the couple pick out a space for the birth pool and instruct how to set it up. It's not rocket science, and my clients are always comfortable when getting ready for a water birth.

As a home birth midwife, I recommend the use of hydrotherapy during the first stage of labor when labor is active and mom is close to the transition stage of labor. Contractions are strong and close together, and laboring moms have to work hard to move through contractions. There is little time between contractions to catch a break from the sensations of labor. When the laboring mom gets into the birth pool, we often hear a sigh of relief with the first contraction she is experiencing while in the pool. The heat of the water changes the sensation of the contractions. The laboring mom usually immediately reports that she enjoys being in the birth pool. Because the water reduces the intensity of contractions, the laboring woman experiences contractions as more manageable.

By offering water birth to my clients, they have the freedom to give birth where they choose. Laboring moms who choose to stay in the water while pushing often give birth in the water. We use a waterproof Doppler so we can easily monitor the baby's heart tones. I encourage the mom to birth her baby into her own hands. When moms feel their babies emerge, they will push carefully and intuitively protect their perineum. When baby is born, moms lift their babies quickly out of the water. Once baby emerges from the water, they often give their first cry.

Some moms are so busy focusing on pushing and working through the sensations in their bodies that they prefer I help with the delivery of their baby.

Water birth is an essential part of my home birth practice. I do believe every woman should have the choice to utilize water in labor. The benefits I have seen in my personal practice are tremendous.

Some women give birth in the water and some choose to give birth out of the water. But the most important part about water birth is that moms have the choice to use water for the labor and/or birth. As a home birth midwife, I am honored to have the experience, knowledge, and understanding of water birth to offer this service to my home birth clients.

PUSHING

When the cervix is fully dilated and baby is low in the pelvis, the body will shift the labor into pushing. As described above, midwives tend to wait for signs from the mom (such as grunting) to indicate that her body is getting ready to push. The urge to push tends to get stronger with every contraction. I encourage mom to listen to her body and work with her body. She resumes whichever position she likes to be in. Many moms choose to lie on their side, some like hands and knees (H+K). Others remain in the birth pool and push in the water. Moms are free to push in any position they desire. We move to listen to baby's heart tones every fifteen minutes at this point in labor. It is common for the woman to change position several times during pushing.

Once baby's head becomes visible, I apply warm compresses on the perineum to help mom cope with the sensations. We encourage mom to start touching baby's head. Some moms want a mirror to see their progress. The excitement in the room becomes palpable. The assistant checks all equipment once more. The blankets are checked to ensure they are warm.

Laboring women tend to listen to their bodies well and just need guidance and encouragement. Midwives typically encourage mom to birth the head slowly to protect her perineum. I encourage mom to push her baby into her own hands. I believe this helps mom to self-direct her pushing effort. At times, the body is delivered in the same contraction as the head. Often the head is born in one contraction and the baby's shoulders and body emerge with the next contraction. I find it important to not rush the actual birthing process. During the final stage of pushing, we listen to baby every other contraction.

As soon as baby is born, baby is handed to mom. I like when moms reach down to catch their own babies. When possible, we have the partner lift baby up into mom's hands.

The first cry is always so special and rewarding. It is always emotional for everyone in the room when baby is born. The birth assistant dries baby off with warm blankets and replaces wet blankets with dry, warm blankets. I encourage my team to avoid talking during this time. This is the family's moment to bond with their new baby.

PLACENTA

Next, we wait for the placenta. Moms are busy meeting their babies, and then, as if transported back in time, they look at me and note "contraction!" It takes a few more contractions and the placenta is born with ease. This process unfolds very easily in due time. We have medications on hand to stop any bleeding or help the placenta along if needed.

Please note that our home birth clients do not routinely have IV access or an IV running. In my practice we have all the equipment to start an IV on hand but only use it as needed—mostly for hydration for first-time moms whose labor is lasting awhile.

The placenta is placed in a bag and put next to mom and baby. We do not cut the cord immediately. The cord, placenta, and baby are one unit. There is no need to clamp and cut immediately. We tend to clamp and cut anywhere from fifteen minutes to one hour after birth and are happy to have partners cut the cord if they desire to do so.

The recovery process begins at this time. Mom's vital signs are checked and her bleeding is closely monitored. The baby's vitals are taken and supervised closely. Baby has not left mom's arms. We are able to take care of the mother-baby unit while they are bonding.

As the new family is bonding, we busy ourselves with cleaning up the birth room. We spend time charting. We prepare food for mom and encourage her to drink plenty of fluid.

NURSING

Newborns are very quickly interested in nursing. They start rooting while lying on mom's chest. On a first baby, we help mom with latching baby. Both mom and baby have great intuition but need some guidance. Seasoned moms just latch baby and let us know that baby is nursing. Most of the babies latch within thirty minutes after birth. Newborns are very alert, eyes wide open and ready for life outside the womb.

PERINEUM

Once the initial excitement of birth is over and baby is settled at the breast, we take a look at mom's vagina.

The most common laceration we see is a first-degree tear, which involves the skin and some tissue along the perineum. When the tissue is approximated well on its own, those tears heal very well without stitches.

If a tear is gaping or deep, or involves muscle, we suture. Lidocaine is applied and the stitches are placed. Mom continues to nurse baby. Besides a few little pricks from the lidocaine, she feels nothing. We see very few deep or complicated lacerations. I contribute this outcome to the healthy nutrition of our moms, intuitive pushing, and the choice of birth position.

In the home birth model of care, the mother and her partner are supported and loved, informed about their choices in childbirth, and encouraged to trust the process. Babies are watched carefully. When labor and birth are not interfered with, it unfolds normally and peacefully.

Women and their partners who choose to have a baby through the home birth model of care are not compromising the health and safety of mom and baby while giving birth. They are making an informed decision to choose a different model of care where they are an active participant in their experience.

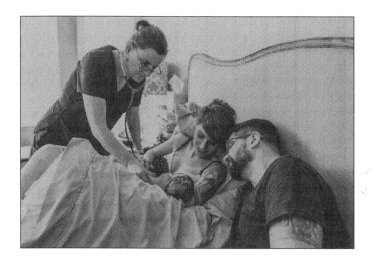

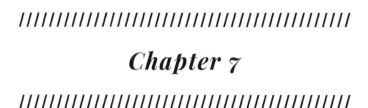

Chapter 7

Your Postpartum Care with a Midwife

One of the most overlooked benefits of home birth? Recovery at home! The mom who has just given birth at home does not have to up and go somewhere. Home birth midwives come to you instead.

AMY'S AND LISA'S POSTPARTUM STORY

Let's visit Amy and Lisa one last time to explore their postpartum experience.

Amy had a beautiful hospital birth. She was able to hold her baby for about ten minutes before baby was moved to the warmer across the room. The nurses assessed her newborn son in the warmer. They measured and weighed him. Then, they applied erythromycin ointment to his eyes and injected vitamin K and hepatitis B vaccine per hospital policy.

Baby boy was wrapped in a blanket, given a clean bill of health, and returned to his mother. She was watching from across the room as her baby was getting his assessment. Dad was right by his side.

Meanwhile, the doctor was busy suturing Amy's perineum for a very common second-degree tear. Her epidural still gave her relief for the suturing and was turned off afterwards. Amy had a blood pressure cuff on her arm that inflated every fifteen minutes to monitor her vitals. She received a routine Pitocin infusion through her IV to prevent bleeding. Once the doctor finished suturing, the nurse gave her a sponge bath. The bed was put back together. She was covered and her baby boy was returned to her arms.

She was so happy to hold her firstborn son and looked forward to nursing him. The nurse helped her get baby latched. Eventually, people left the room, lights were turned off, and mom and baby were alone for a few minutes.

After several hours, the epidural catheter was taken out.

Amy was moved to her recovery room via wheelchair. The room was much smaller than the birth room. She would be in the postpartum unit until she was discharged home from the hospital.

The two days Amy spent on the postpartum unit felt like a blur. Her room was a revolving door of hospital staff. There was a nurse to take care of baby, a nurse to take care of her, a pediatrician checking on baby, the ob-gyn checking on her, a lactation consultant, people who were filing the birth certificate, technicians who were checking the baby's hearing and oxygen levels, and nurse's aides coming in and out of the room at all hours of the day and night. And then there were her friends and family who stopped by to congratulate her and meet the new baby. She was able to sneak in some naps, but otherwise did not get much rest.

At discharge, she was told to follow up with her ob-gyn at six weeks postpartum. The baby would need to see the pediatrician within two days of birth.

Amy was happy to return home. She took her son to the pediatrician at two days old and two weeks old. He was thriving and growing well. Amy was recovering too. She didn't receive her first checkup until six weeks later; at the routine postpartum visit with her ob-gyn. Amy had many questions about nursing, her body, and her emotions. She found many answers online. Amy did not want to come across as insecure and wanted to make sure she looked competent. She was fully dressed every day, did not stay down much, hosted her visitors, and kept her emotions secret.

LISA'S POSTPARTUM STORY

Lisa had a beautiful home birth. Her baby stayed in her arms for two hours, nursing for a full hour before falling fast asleep. While nursing, her husband fed her homemade food that she had prepared the day before. The midwife numbed her perineum with lidocaine and placed a few sutures. Lisa was not even aware of the suturing. She was too busy bonding with and staring at her new baby.

After a few hours, Lisa felt the need to get up and go to the bathroom. The assistant midwife helped her, holding her arm to ensure she was stable. The other midwife made the bed while baby rested in dad's arms. Lisa wanted to shower, so the midwife assisted her and stayed close by. The shower felt glorious. She put on a new gown and walked back to a freshly made bed.

The midwife started the newborn exam after Lisa settled back into bed. The baby was right next to her the entire time. She watched the exam closely. Baby was weighed, measured, and carefully evaluated. Lisa told the midwife that she wanted the baby to have the vitamin K injection (to help prevent bleeding), but declined the erythromycin ointment and was planning to get the hepatitis B vaccine later from the pediatrician. The midwife administered the vitamin K as discussed and handed baby back to mom.

The baby latched onto Lisa's breast again. The midwives packed equipment, worked on laundry, and gave instructions for mom and baby to Lisa and her husband. The midwife was planning to call in a few hours and scheduled a home visit for the next day. Hugs were exchanged and the midwives quietly left the house. Lisa and her husband chatted a bit longer before drifting off to sleep in their own familiar bed. The baby was resting next to them in a co-sleeper attached to the bed.

The midwives returned to check on both Lisa and baby several times during the first week. At week two, they were seen in office. Lisa's vital signs were recorded at every visit, her bleeding was evaluated, any new feelings and emotions were discussed, and she was given nursing support.

At each visit, the baby was weighed and his vitals checked. The midwives performed a heel stick to collect blood for the newborn metabolic screening and gave a referral for the newborn hearing screen. The paperwork to file the birth certificate was collected. Lisa was encouraged to stay home, rest, and nurse baby only. Her questions were answered. Her roller coaster of emotions was addressed. She felt very supported and loved. Baby was thriving and doing well. Lisa started seeing the pediatrician at two weeks postpartum. She had her final checkup with her midwife at six weeks postpartum. Lisa was very sad to say goodbye to her midwife. She had become a trusted companion, whom Lisa was fond of.

IMMEDIATE POSTPARTUM RECOVERY

Mom recovers in her own bed surrounded by family, friends, and the midwife team. The first two hours are spent nursing, bonding, eating, and being pampered.

We offer mom over-the-counter Advil or Tylenol for any discomfort she experiences. Most women take a dose of Advil or Tylenol; some decline any pain reliever. It never ceases to impress everyone how mom—who was in the throes of labor only moments before—is smiling, talking, and simply being herself immediately after giving birth.

The mom's bleeding, blood pressure, pulse, and temperature are checked frequently during the postpartum recovery period. The newborn's lungs, breathing rate, heart rate, temperature, and color are checked frequently during this time as well. We keep a close eye on both mom and baby without disrupting the bonding process. All of our tasks are easily accomplished while baby is nursing.

A few hours after giving birth, moms are ready to get up and walk to the bathroom. This is the first time baby leaves mom's arms. Baby is placed in her partner's arms. The woman walks to the bathroom, empties her bladder, and sponges off or takes a shower. One of the midwives accompanies her, assisting when needed. The other midwife removes the birth layer of sheets from the bed. A second set of sheets, on which mom will recover, is revealed. Mom returns to a freshly made bed.

NEWBORN EXAM

Midwives are trained and certified to complete newborn exams. The exam is done in bed, right next to mom. We carefully evaluate the baby's physical appearance, listen to heart and lungs, and finally weigh and measure baby. Routine newborn medications such as vitamin K and erythromycin eye ointment are offered. Footprints are done. Cord care is administered.

Mom and her partner watch during the exam. Weighing baby in a little sling is often a favorite photo moment. Parents decide on the first outfit and diaper, or none. Finally, baby is returned to mom for another nursing session.

CLEANING UP AND POSTPARTUM INSTRUCTION

Before leaving, the midwife team removes all equipment, loads the washing machine and dryer, and takes out the trash. My general rule is to leave the house the way I found it, with the exception of a baby in mom's arms.

Parents receive instructions on how to take care of newborn and mom, problems to report, and when to call for concerns.

We exchange hugs and goodbyes, and then leave the home. The couple is tucked into bed, ready to doze off.

POSTPARTUM FOLLOW-UP CARE

New mothers are encouraged to "lie in," meaning stay down in the bed or on a couch, rest, sleep, and nurse baby. During the first week, mom's only responsibility is to take care of her own hygiene needs, bond with and nurse baby, eat, hydrate rest, and sleep.

In my practice, I return on day one and day three postpartum. Mom then comes to my office around one and a half weeks after birth. Mom and baby are considered a unit and are followed together. Each visit is at least one and a half hours, and often two hours long. I'm often overheard saying, "If we get week one right, we are off to a great start."

During postpartum visits, proper nursing techniques are established, confidence with nursing is built, realistic expectations for body changes are discussed, mom's confidence is bolstered, emotions are discussed, the birth experience is processed, and much more. I check in daily via text and phone in the first week, once more in week two. My statistics reveal that 100 percent of my clients breastfeed at six weeks postpartum. Further, my clients successfully transition adding baby to the family.

At the six-week visit, we provide a well-woman exam, discuss birth control, family planning, and emotions. It is a bittersweet visit. The client and midwife have spent almost one year on this journey together. They have grown close and built a strong relationship with each other. The clients are often sad to say goodbye to their midwife until the next pregnancy.

The continued support midwives provide is vital for healthy families.

BREASTFEEDING SUPPORT

Midwives tend to be very committed to helping mothers successfully breastfeed. We encourage pregnant women to learn about breastfeeding during pregnancy. Mom's anatomy for nursing is evaluated during the initial physical exam. Right after baby is born and ready to nurse, the initial latch is fostered. Uninterrupted nursing after birth is the foundation to a successful nursing relationship.

Midwives answer many questions during the first few days after birth. Encouragement is provided, the range of normal is explained, and sore and cracked nipples are evaluated. If there are problems breastfeeding, we refer to a lactation consultant. If specific problems (such as tongue-tie) are suspected, we refer to a specialist for further evaluation.

Baby is weighed frequently in the first week to monitor weight gain, and parents are encouraged to record baby's output (urine and stools) to help screen for any nursing or milk-supply problems.

I always tell my clients you only recover after birth once, or perhaps a handful of times. As I midwife, I help recover clients at least two to three times per month and have done so hundreds of times in total. In the first week after birth, every day is different—physically and emotionally—for mom. She needs lots of support and encouragement for this period. Midwives have mastered the art of recovering families post-birth.

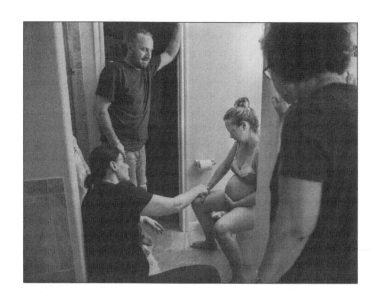

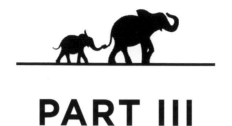

PART III

Getting Started with a Midwife

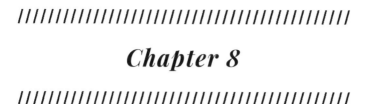

Chapter 8

//

So You're Ready to Take Charge of Your Birth

HOW DO I FIND A HOME BIRTH MIDWIFE?

Give yourself the opportunity to meet a home birth midwife!

Step one is to find out if midwifery is legal in your state. Next go online and start your midwife search, use key search terms like "home birth," "water birth," or "mid-wives." Reviewing the websites of home birth midwives gives you great insight into different personalities and practice styles. From there, I recommend contacting two to three midwives to schedule in-person interviews.

Those consultations are free and you will learn a lot by talking to a midwife.

Each midwife is unique. They vary in philosophies and practice styles. It is important to meet several midwives to see who feels right for you. The connection you feel to your home birth midwife is the foundation on which you'll build your relationship.

TEN QUESTIONS TO ASK A HOME BIRTH MIDWIFE

1. What is your midwifery philosophy and practice style?
2. What is your education, training, certification, and experience level?
3. What do your home birth services include and exclude?
4. What are your testing and treatment options?
5. What connections to related professionals or hospitals do you have for genetic testing, sonograms, co-care, transfer of care, pregnancy support, classes, and bodywork?
6. Who is on your team and when will I meet them?
7. What are the limitations on when I can give birth at home (i.e. weeks of gestation)?
8. What are your/your team's qualifications for emergencies? What emergency medications do you carry?
9. Are you comfortable with water birth?

10. What are your personal practice statistics on hospital transfer? What are the reasons for transfer of care to the hospital?

This list of questions should reveal great information to you in order to make a decision to move forward with the midwife you are meeting.

I think meeting a home birth midwife belongs on everyone's bucket list. They are extraordinary human beings who have spent their time devoted to serving women and families.

Go! Contact a home birth midwife today!

THE COST

Remember Amy and Lisa? We're not finished with them quite yet! As a reminder, Amy chose the medical model of care (and a hospital birth). Lisa chose the midwifery model of care (and a home birth).

Both Amy and Lisa had uneventful births and feel good about the care they received through the two representative models.

Let's look at the cost for each model.

AMY'S COST

Amy had health insurance through her employer. She had a deductible of $3,000 and 80/20 coverage for everything after her deductible. This means that Amy is 100 percent responsible for all healthcare expenses up to $3,000. For everything over $3,000, Amy pays 20 percent of all expenses out of pocket and her insurance covers the rest.

The total cost for Amy's prenatal care, birth, and one postpartum visit from her ob-gyn—called a "global fee"— was $3,000. This was all paid out of pocket, as she had not yet reached her deductible.

In addition, Amy received a bill from the lab, the hospital for her birth, a bill from the anesthesiologist for the epidural, and a bill from the pediatrician. Together, these invoices totaled another $10,000. Since she had met her deductible, her insurance covered 80 percent of the bill ($8,000), and Amy was responsible for 20 percent of the bill ($2,000). In the end, Amy paid a grand total of $5,000 out of pocket for prenatal, birth, and postpartum care.

LISA'S COST

Like Amy, Lisa also had insurance through her employer. She had a $2,000 deductible.

Lisa's health insurance did not cover home birth, so she

opted to utilize the home birth midwife's private pay plan of $4,000. This fee covered all prenatal care, the birth, and several postpartum visits. She made seven payments of $571 to the midwife during her prenatal period. She utilized her insurance to pay for her sonogram and lab tests for which she had to pay $500 out of pocket. By the time she went into labor, all bills for prenatal care, birth care, and postpartum recovery were paid. She would not receive another bill from her midwife as she had prepaid with the midwives' cash payment plan of $4,000.

COST OF BIRTH UNDER THE MEDICAL MODEL OF CARE

Lacie Glover describes the cost of childbirth in the US in her article published on NerdWallet:

> According to data from the US Department of Health and Human Services for 2014, the latest year available, national median charges for childbirth hospital stays in the US were:
>
> - $13,524 for delivery and care for mothers.
> - $3,660 for newborns.
>
> Most hospitals use a fee-for-service system in which each test, visit, procedure, and consultation is billed separately. The facility fee, or hospital charge, and the charge for the

delivering physician make up a large portion of costs for many uncomplicated deliveries.

Aside from the hospital charge and the doctors' fees, costs typically include lab tests, epidural, radiology, and any medications provided.[3]

Birthing your baby in the hospital involves many practitioners with various qualifications. Your ob-gyn or nurse-midwife provides the prenatal care, birth, immediate follow-up in the hospital, and one visit at six weeks postpartum. A hospital birth involves the hospital and the costs associated with its services. The anesthesiologist charges for services rendered. The pediatrician, who takes care of baby in the hospital and after baby is released from the hospital, charges for care provided to baby. These costs add up. Please keep in mind that a C-section increases the cost of birth dramatically.

Women and their partners often pay significantly into their health insurance plans in the form of monthly premiums and would like to utilize this coverage. Medical providers and hospitals are "in-network" with many insurance plans. Depending on a plan's individual ben-

---

3   Lacie Glover, "How Much Does It Cost to Have a Baby?" NerdWallet,
     February 27, 2017, https://www.nerdwallet.com/blog/health/medical-costs/
     how-much-does-it-cost-to-have-a-baby/.

efits, the medical model of care tends to be covered under most insurance plans.

Despite the fact that childbirth is often covered by the individual plan, it is important to understand that the medical model of care is expensive and costs can easily add up. Further, it is very important that you know your deductible and what percentage of healthcare expenses (if any) you are responsible for after the deductible is met. Over the last few years, deductibles have increased, and today, 40 percent of Americans have "high deductible" plans.

COST OF BIRTH UNDER THE MIDWIFERY MODEL OF CARE

Predominately, home birth midwives do not accept insurance or only accept limited types of insurance.

The reason is simple. Home birth is often not covered by insurance and/or the midwife credentials are not recognized. Further, midwives typically carry a very small patient load, and thus, most insurance companies will not credential them as in-network providers. Reimbursement for an out-of-network provider is just a fraction of what an in-network provider receives.

In my midwifery practice, I have always worked with

insurance companies when applicable. I use an insurance billing company. We start with a "verification of benefits" and move forward by discussing benefits available. Recently, I have seen more "verifications of benefits" that cover my credential as a CPM, benefits available for home birth, and the flexibility to file a one-time "in-network exception."

The majority of home birth midwives offer services via a private-pay global fee. This fee generally includes all prenatal care, the birth, birth assistant, postpartum care, and any home visits. The baby is included in the care up to six weeks postpartum.

The included services and global fee vary based on geographic location. The cost ranges anywhere from $3,000 to $6,000 and is often due around the thirty-sixth week of pregnancy.

Home birth midwives offer payment plans, take credit cards, and at times, barter.

The global fee generally covers the midwife's services only. Labs and sonogram fees are excluded, but are typically covered by insurance. For clients without insurance, I offer labs at drastically discounted prices.

I think it's a fair statement that midwives are very affordable for the comprehensive and compassionate care they provide. We are on call 24/7 and spend at least one hour with our clients per visit. At times, we labor with our clients for days, only to turn around and provide excellent postpartum follow-up for mom and baby.

The best way I can convey this value is through the story of a first-time mom who hired me shortly before Thanksgiving. She said that she and her husband relayed all the services that were included in my home birth package to a large group at the Thanksgiving table. They then asked the group to guess the cost. Answers included $10,000, $15,000, and beyond. Far from it, my friends; far from it!

HOW TO TALK TO FAMILY MEMBERS ABOUT HOME BIRTH

If you're reading this book, you've likely done a great deal of research on home birth and are considering having your baby at home. However, you can't assume that everyone else has done the same.

Family members worry about safety, money, and outcomes. Before dismissing the idea of home birth, it is important to understand what home birth actually looks like with a qualified midwife and how prenatal care and postpartum care are actually done. Understanding the midwifery model of care is vital in order to have a conversation with a skeptical family member.

Explore the concerns and fears of the skeptical family member. Are these fears based on beliefs around home birth that are not compatible with today's reality? Or are they concerns based on something entirely different? I find that most people are skeptical based on their understanding and thoughts of home birth, which do not compare to the actual reality of care with a licensed, skilled midwife.

Safety is most likely what comes to mind. Meeting a home birth midwife and using the interview questions outlined above is a great way to start the process. Bring your skeptical family member to the interview.

THE SKEPTICAL PARTNER

It is not uncommon for a woman to want a home birth but find that her partner is very skeptical or concerned about this model of care.

The statistics enclosed in this book are a great place to start in debunking safety concerns. The next step is to research midwives and meet two to three midwives that appear to be a good fit.

Another common concern is financial. Most people think

that birth in a hospital is routinely covered. This is far from reality. There are many hidden costs associated with birth. The partner who is worried about cost should research the cost associated with prenatal care, birth in the hospital, postpartum care, and expenses related to newborn care. This can be tedious but give great insight. Please refer to the section on the cost of midwifery. Home birth is very affordable with no hidden price tags attached.

Again, social conditioning and our emotions influence our decision about where to give birth. Encourage your skeptical partner to look into his concerns and meet a midwife.

THE SKEPTICAL FAMILY

You and your partner may have agreed on home birth as a great choice for birthing your baby. You bring your decision to your extended family and they may have questions.

COMMON QUESTIONS: WHAT IF...

1. The baby has the cord wrapped around its neck?
    A. Babies commonly have the cord around their necks. This is easily managed by the midwife. The cord is reduced as baby is being born. If baby is affected by the cord compression, we hear this with the Doppler when we listen to baby's heart

tones. Plans are made to transfer care or prepare to manage the birth at home. In my experience, this is rarely a problem.

2. She's bleeding too much?
   B. Midwives are trained to manage bleeding and carry medications to help stop bleeding. They can stop bleeding, stabilize mom, and transfer to a hospital if appropriate. We see very little bleeding in home birth.

3. She wants pain relief after all?
   C. Women can change their minds during a home birth. If this happens, we transfer mom to the hospital to birth baby and receive pain relief. We see this scenario rarely.

4. She needs a C-section? All our friends, and even her sister, had C-sections.
   D. The national C-section rate is 32 percent. The home birth midwife C-section rate is 5 percent. The World Health Organization has long stated that the average C-section rate should be between 10 and 15 percent. Midwives do not interfere in the birthing process but do transfer to hospital if problems develop. Interventions such as Pitocin induction before babies are due and Pitocin augmentation during labor lead to a 60 percent

chance of C-section for a first-time mom delivering in a hospital. As midwives, we wait for baby to be born. We transfer if we have concerns during the labor and birthing process.

5. The baby is big? We have big babies in our family.
   E. Midwives consider 8.5 pounds to 9.5 pounds a normal-size baby and are comfortable delivering larger babies. We monitor weight gain and nutrition carefully. When a woman is able to move freely and birth freely, she tends not to have a problem with the size of the baby. If a baby is overgrown and not fitting in the pelvis, we transfer care to the hospital with our non-emergent protocol and continue the birth in the hospital.

6. Something goes wrong?
   F. This question is very encompassing. Midwives are trained and able to detect problems during the pregnancy, birth, and postpartum. As a matter of fact, that is what you hire a licensed midwife for. She is supervising the pregnancy, birth, and postpartum. Her job is to detect variations outside the range of normal and work on returning to the range of normal. If she is unable to do so, she utilizes help from the medical system or related professionals. Midwives are trained to stabilize and transfer either mom or baby in medical emer-

gencies. They carry medication and equipment to do so and continue to train for emergency scenarios.

In my experience, once many of the misconceptions around home birth are debunked, extended family tends to be very supportive.

As a woman, it is important to remember that this is your body, your pregnancy, and your birth. You are becoming a mother, whether it is for the first time or subsequent times, and you are on your own journey. Support for a home birth from family members is rewarding but not critical. If your heart desires a home birth and your partner is supportive, then you get to choose whether to write your own birth story or to please your family.

//

Chapter 9

//

Birth Stories by My Clients

AMELIA'S FIRST BIRTH—FIRST HOME BIRTH

I didn't think I would ever get to be a mom. After years of bad relationships, I had resigned myself to being the cool aunt. But then I met my husband, and he changed my world. Six years later, we decided to start trying for our first baby. We were extremely lucky and conceived on our first try. I was thrilled to tears and really nervous.

Then the morning (read: all-day) sickness hit. I believe some of my heavy sickness was likely anxiety that was so intense I was literally sick with worry. But my personality tells me that when I'm worried the most, I need to plan. So I went about planning my pregnancy. I knew full well that I couldn't control much of what my body did, but I was determined to control every external factor that I could. So I began researching techniques and doctors and procedures and so on. As a result, Netflix suggested I start watching *Call the Midwife*, and as creeped out as I am that technology watches me so closely, I am so glad it did. I watched woman after woman have amazing relationships with their midwives. Relationships that survived the births of multiple children, struggles with fertility, challenges with postpartum depression, various health issues, and well—everything. These midwives were in it for a deeper purpose than delivering babies—they wanted to empower women. They helped so many women to be healthy and safe, and really guided them through what I (correctly) assumed would be the toughest journey in the world—becoming "mom." So I watched and studied and went to my ten-minute-long doctor appointments, and all was great.

Finally, it was time for the hospital tour! I started asking nurses about how it is my doctor makes all the births for the women in her practice and whhhoooaaa, wait a minute, she does not! What? But how? You mean to tell me that all the obstetricians in the practice (four) are on a rotation, and I have a 75 percent chance of delivering with a doctor that I really don't know AT ALL? Wow. I was in shock. How could I have missed this? THIS did not help with the worry. Then, as if being guided to a different option, I started reading hospital birth stories. Stories of women who are told not to push, even though their bodies scream to do differently, or babies whisked away to gather vitals instead of getting immediate skin-to-skin. And mothers not being allowed to eat while getting the longest and most intense workout of their life. These were the tame stories. To say I was horrified is an understatement. I remember thinking, "Wow, I wish I could deliver my baby like they did in *Call the Midwife.*" Enter Google. Oh my gosh, I CAN. So I'm nearly twenty weeks at this point, and nervous to change my plan, when my husband ever so casually says, "Oh, that would be great. I was born with a midwife at home, too." Well, I'm determined now—because I just know if my mother-in-law can do it, then I can, too. I research what to look for in a midwife, research cost, research how to interview them, read reviews, and end up in contact with Monika. Of my top three choices, she was the only one with a spot open—because midwives only take as many clients as they can reasonably handle—another comforting detail to hear! So I prepared my questionnaire, drove down, and our first meeting was ah-mazing. She was in no rush, she loved to talk, she didn't float me any nonsense, and she was realistic and honest, while being compassionate and genuinely interested in any aspect of my life that affected my pregnancy. I was hooked. My entire heart knew—she was the one. I kid you not—I was more confident picking her as my midwife than I was marrying my husband. I honestly looked forward to my checkups, and by the time my delivery arrived I felt fully prepared, calm, and confident. One of the steps I have taken, at the suggestion of Monika, was to read *Birthing from Within*. Through all the activities, I was sure that Monika would deliver my baby, it would be dark out, I would deliver in bed, and Liam would come a few days earlier than when he was due. She also suggested hypnobirthing, and after independently researching the course, I fell in love with the idea. The meditation and affirmations were amazing at lowering my anxiety and my blood pressure and raising my confidence.

It was at the last appointment before my due date that I walked in and Monika said, "You look very heavy with baby," and for the first time, I felt a little heavy with baby! I went home knowing it would be soon, but not too anxious because I also knew that first-time moms usually deliver later, when boom—my water broke! I immediately called Monika and we laughed at how glad we were I chose not to have a pelvic exam earlier that day. My contractions started about twenty-three hours later, after lots of walking, a little fooling around, and just before the time where she was going to suggest I head to a hospital to get labor started. Every call with Monika was wild to me because she could tell when I was having a contraction before I even knew! She showed up a few hours later, and I was dilated to seven centimeters. That poor woman walked in at the height of my really loud contractions (I'm a yeller, ha ha) and was so calm, just reminding me to breathe. I don't remember much over the next few hours, other than moving from bed to toilet to bath to sink (and so on) to change my laboring positions. The hypnobirthing techniques were great, as they took me to what Monika called "Labor Land," and it made the hours pass like minutes. But I do remember pushing so hard in the bath and just knowing I wasn't doing it right. Monika helped me to the bed and brought in a birthing stool, which helped me find the correct muscles—from which I had almost immediate success. I lay back on the bed and soon after birthed my son while lying on my side, with my husband in front of me and Monika right beside me. My son was immediately laid on my chest, and while he breathed gently and seemed incredibly calm, he wouldn't even cry until we slapped his feet a little a few minutes later. I think the birth was so peaceful that when he arrived, he was just relaxed and happy. (Side note—all of my visions of delivery from *Birthing from Within* were accurate!)

I have literally never been happier in my life than when I first held my son. He was the most perfect thing I had ever seen, and my heart was exploding with love. I remember crying so hard because I loved him so much that it was almost painful. After I finally was able to come down off cloud nine, I let him do the breast crawl, and Monika and Deb (Monika's partner) helped me make sure he had a perfect latch. They did all the vitals, cleaned up, and headed out. I fed my son and we all laid down to rest. My husband fell asleep immediately, and I just lay there looking in absolute wonder at the most perfect person I had ever seen. My delivery had gone swimmingly. I felt calm, safe, happy, and especially relaxed being in the comfort of my own home with midwives I trusted.

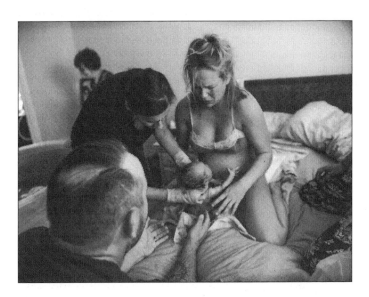

SARAH'S THIRD BIRTH—FIRST HOME BIRTH

James was my first home birth after experiencing two hospital births with my first- born children who were twins and my second born. The first hospital birth had been a twin birth and it was a huge ordeal delivering in the operating room with a large number of doctors, nurses, and students—most of whom I had never met. My second pregnancy and delivery was uneventful compared to the twin birth. I have been blessed to have very healthy pregnancies, and as a result, I did not feel like I was given the personal care and attention that I was desiring for my second birth since everything was so smooth and easy. The second birth was a standard hospital birth with very little interaction from my doctor. With both of these deliveries, I did have a hard time with the insertion of the epidurals that honestly frightened me. So with pregnancy number three, I was looking for a more natural experience that was personal, caring, and allowed me to have my baby in the privacy of my home surrounded by people who cared for me and were genuinely concerned for my welfare and that of my baby.

After being so happy with the care that I received from my midwives during my third pregnancy, I began anticipating the birth of my fourth child. Having no previous experience with labor pains or even pre-labor pains, I did not know what to expect labor-wise as my due date approached. Beginning the night of my due date, I was very anxious and got little sleep. Contractions plagued me off and on in the night, and I remember calling my midwife to talk with her about my symptoms. She was able to evaluate my condition over the phone and prescribe some remedies, and labor pains ceased after a time. The following night was a replay of the night before. Night three was different. The contractions were more intense and more frequent. My anxiety was high after calling my midwife two nights in a row, but on the other hand, I was also anxious to get my midwives to my house before labor intensified.

About four in the morning, my midwives decided the time had come for them to head to my house. It is strange how your mind can control your body so readily. I was still anxious, wondering if I had called them at the right time. By the time they arrived, the contractions had stalled and I was lying in the bed feeling so guilty and stressed about the whole situation. Their gentle words and care reassured me that I had called them at the appropriate time. I was so thankful for their kind words and calm demeanor. I was given some homeopathic tablets to help ease the anxiety and relax so that labor could return. I lay in bed for a few hours as my midwives sat together outside enjoying the sunrise. I remember watching them visit together and being so thankful that they were at my home ready to support me when my body was ready.

At nine in the morning, I was sent on a walk with my husband down our county road. While we walked, the midwives prepared the room and bed for birth. The walk was all my body needed, and labor pains began to intensify. I knew then that this was the day my baby would be born. I had questioned myself all morning until that hour when the rushes came one after the other, each one becoming more intense. This being my first labor, I did not welcome the rushes the way that I wish I had. It was a struggle to get through the pains. I was encouraged by the midwives to immerse myself in the bathtub for a while. The water was helpful and a nice change. After a time, we moved to my room, and then the kitchen, where I could stand and sway while holding on to my husband or a chair. I was so thankful for my midwives' support and guidance through this intense physical experience.

Early afternoon, the decision was made to break my water. It was explained to me that my sac was very thick and tight, like a balloon. The sac was keeping me from progressing any further, so I did not mind a little help to quickly further things along. I remember the labor pains and pressure intensifying tremendously once my water was broken. I sat paralyzed on the floor on all fours as each rush came, giving me very little rest time before the next one occurred. Baby was near!

Around forty-five minutes after breaking my water, it was time to push. I was not prepared for this experience and the sensations that followed. Pushing the baby out was very intense and with these new feelings and sensations, fear gripped me again. My husband held me down as I tried to push myself off the other side of the bed, even at one time kicking because I did not know how to respond as the baby's head began to immerge. My midwives were very calm yet firm about what I needed to do to push my baby out. Within a few minutes, my son, James, was born. Oh, how happy I was but so exhausted. I held him close as my midwives examined my situation and I could tell they were in an intense mode, but I did not know why. They quickly explained to me that I needed a shot of Pitocin to stop my bleeding. After a few minutes, another shot was given. My husband and I still talk about how we were both in awe at that time over their quick response and wisdom as they worked through the situation.

A few minutes passed, and I was told that it was time to push out the placenta. I remember laughing a little inside and thinking to myself, "I don't have a single ounce of energy left to push that placenta out." I voiced my thoughts and my midwife explained how much easier it is to push out the placenta than the baby. She was right. Thank goodness the placenta is a soft tissue. I found out later, after the rush of the delivery had passed, that my midwives examined the entire placenta thoroughly. They were both surprised at how healthy and thick my placenta had been and they credited the health of the placenta and the health of the baby to a very healthy organic diet. Their words are still an encouragement to me today to maintain healthy eating habits, especially in pregnancy.

My midwives stayed another hour or two, caring for my baby, my husband, and me. They did all the washing of the sheets, helped prepare food to nourish my husband and me, and kept a close eye on baby James. I felt so nurtured and loved. They left us tucked into bed with clean sheets, full bellies, and a peace, knowing we had the entire night to ourselves. No one was going to force their way into my room at two in the morning to take my blood pressure or take baby's temperature or tell me it was time to nurse. My husband and I were the ones to make all the decisions in the comfort of our home with our baby, and we couldn't have been happier about that.

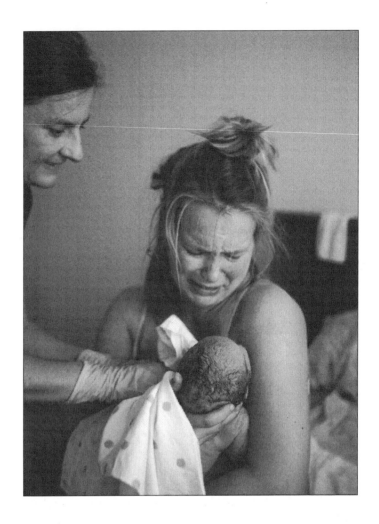

ANNE'S THIRD BIRTH—FIRST HOME BIRTH

My first daughter was a planned home birth that ended in a hospital transfer due to "failure to progress." I woke up at forty-one weeks and five days to my water breaking, but I never went into active labor. After thirty-six hours and only progressing to four centimeters, she was born via C-section. My son's birth was a redemptive VBAC at a birth center with wonderful midwives and a chiropractor who saved me from a second caesarian. His birth also began with my water breaking (at forty-one weeks). It was a slow start, almost identical to my daughter's, but after seventeen hours of almost no progress, I received an adjustment, which put him in the right position. My labor went full tilt almost immediately, and he was in my arms three hours later! We moved to Texas in 2017 and decided to wait until we felt the timing was right before trying for another baby. In February of 2018, I got a very big surprise the day before my birthday in the form of two pink lines! I happened to learn that I was pregnant a few hours before I hopped on a flight for Vegas, but that's a story for another time. I hadn't decided how I wanted to deliver this time around and considered just going the "normal" route with my ob-gyn in the hospital. But after two appointments with him and learning I would be considered "high risk" because of my age and cae-sarian history (and thus limited on my laboring options), I decided I would try to achieve the home birth I had set out for five years earlier. Being new to the area, I wasn't sure who I should use as my midwife, until I came across Monika's website. It was a Sunday afternoon, and I defi-nitely did not expect her to answer when I called, but she did (midwives have no office hours). We ended up talking for almost an hour, and I knew that she was exactly who I needed to help bring my baby earth side!

Since my two previous pregnancies had both gone post-date, it was no surprise when I woke up on the morning of week forty-one still pregnant. The night before, I had asked Monika if she would feel comfortable sweeping my membranes and trying some natural methods of induction to help move things along. She agreed and said she would be over the next morning. But before she even arrived, I had my first sign that labor was nearing—I lost my mucus plug. This hadn't happened with my two previous labors, so I was excited to know that my body was already doing work. When she got to my home, she did a check and I was about two centimeters. She did the sweep, and I took some homeopathic tinctures, walked, and did breast pumping for a few hours. I was having strong Braxton-Hicks contractions but couldn't say that they felt like labor yet. Monika decided to leave for a little while to give me some time to relax and see if my body would "tip over" and start labor. Before she left, she checked me once more and found I was at a solid three centimeters. This was encouraging, since I had never dilated that much before my water breaking. We went about our evening as usual; I made dinner and got the kids ready for bed, all while having intermittent mild contractions about ten minutes apart. They weren't getting stronger or more intense, so I didn't really think anything was happening. My parents live on the same property as we do and had offered to take the kids for the night "just in case," which was such a huge blessing to not have to worry about them. I talked to Monika after sending the kids next door around eight o'clock; she told me to relax and we would reassess in the morning. My husband and I watched a movie and my contractions spaced out even further. They were now fifteen to twenty minutes apart. I was a disappointed that we had done all of that work earlier in the day only to have things fizzle out. About eleven o'clock, we went to bed. I had been lying down for maybe five minutes when I had a strong contraction. It was much more intense than what I had been experiencing during the day. For the next hour, my husband and I timed the contractions and waited to see if they would slow down. They didn't. I called Monika at midnight and told her things were picking up. She said she would get on the road right away. We also called my mom to let her know what was happening so she could join us.

Monika arrived at my house an hour later. When she arrived, I was still walking around and in fact managed to put on a pot of coffee for her and the team that would be coming soon, but things were starting to intensify. I remember having a contraction in the kitchen that put me on my knees and thinking, "Okay, it's really happening." Monika asked if she could check my cervix. I didn't think the contractions I had been having earlier were doing much, but to my shock, I was already at five centimeters! I was so excited to hear that news. I was halfway there!

Monika suggested that I get into the tub and labor there while she got set up and called the rest of the team to come. I have to add this in—I've always heard that getting into the tub too early can potentially stall out labor, so when she suggested I get in, I was a little skeptical. I thought, it's too early! I hadn't been in labor long enough! I shouldn't be getting in yet; what if things slow down? HA! Things did NOT slow down, but they did feel about a million times better in the hot water. I labored in the tub for around an hour, but soon started feeling really nauseous. *Bonus husband points for holding a trash can for your wife to get sick in!* This was new for me, as I had never gotten sick during labor before. I knew it is usually a sign of transition but I was in total denial because I had only been having painful contractions for less than two hours. I got out of the tub and decided to labor on the toilet for a while. I had done this during my son's labor and if there was one bit of advice I could give to moms during birth, it would be to get on the toilet. It puts you and baby in such a great position and allows you to "labor down," and less pushing time is a good time! Then I moved to the bed and tried to find a comfortable position, but that just wasn't going to happen. These were the hardest contractions of the labor. I can remember lying on my side with Monika lying facing toward me, speaking calming words; my husband kneeling next to the bed, rubbing my back; and my doula at the end of the bed, massaging my feet. The contractions were right on top of one another, and I felt like I couldn't even catch my breath between them. I really struggled to relax during them and found myself arching up and squeezing a washcloth as hard as I could as they hit. I don't know how long I was on the bed; this part of labor gets a little fuzzy. They say you "go inside yourself," and this is exactly what was happening. I could see things going on around me, but it was like I was in a different realm. Thankfully, soon after, I started to feel "pushy." I felt my body wanting to bear down, but my mind couldn't comprehend that it was time yet. I got up and went to the bathroom again. I felt the most relief in that position and the urge to push got stronger. Monika encouraged me to listen to my body and so I began to put force behind the urges. After a few contractions, there was a loud "POP" and my water broke! Another benefit of laboring on the toilet: no mess! At this point, I heard Monika say to me "Okay, time to get off the toilet; we don't want baby to come out there," but I couldn't quite bring myself to move yet. I stayed there through a few more contractions and then finally mustered up the determination to get back on the bed. I tried pushing on hands and knees (this was the position I delivered my son in), but I couldn't seem to get any "traction" and felt my pushing wasn't doing much. Then I tried pushing while lying on my side and finally wound up on my back, with my husband helping to prop me up. I felt Rose moving down during these pushes and soon I could reach down and feel her head. By this point I was DONE with labor and ready to get this girl out, during the next contraction she crowned and without waiting for another one, I pushed again and she was HERE! Rose Evelyn Faith came out pink and squalling and perfect at 4:06 a.m. (FOUR HOURS after I called Monika) November 11, 2018, seven pounds, twelve ounces and 20.5 inches long.

It is so incredible how you can go from the most intense pain you've ever experienced to pure joy and relief in a matter of seconds, and that is exactly what happens in those last moments of labor. There was such a beautiful presence that filled the room the moment she was born. It was sacred and emotional and above all PEACEFUL. I brought her to my chest and we all rejoiced in the wonder of the new life we had been blessed with. My husband holding me and my mom standing close by, happy tears were shed by all. The postpartum activity was purposeful but unhurried and my husband and I relaxed on the bed as Monika and team completed their tasks. After a short time, my mom went next door and woke up my daughter. She was able to meet her baby sister minutes after she arrived and witness her mother during her strongest moment. She was beaming as she held "her baby." Monika and her team stayed with us a couple more hours to ensure all was well with Rose and me, then they were ready to be on their way. They tucked us into bed, said goodbye, and left us to rest with our sweet girl.

The home birth I had longed for, for five years had happened! It happened quickly, it happened peacefully, and it happened without fear! It was one of the most incredible experiences of my life. Yes, there was pain and intensity, but it was overwhelmingly beautiful, spiritual, and life-changing. I'm so thankful that God allowed me to experience birth this way and that He brought Monika into my life to guide me through it!

The above story refers to VBAC (vaginal birth after cesarean section), which is, statistically, a risk factor for emergency complications of labor. Some VBAC patients have less risk, such as women who have already had a vaginal birth. However, whether a home birth is still an option, is an important discussion that must occur between the midwife and patient when a patient has or develops risk factors of pregnancy.

KRISTEN'S FIRST BIRTH—FIRST HOME BIRTH

Even though we liked our ob-gyn, Anthony and I decided that we wanted a home birth for our baby. Monika and Debra helped me finally figure out a solution to my around-the-clock morning sickness. I felt educated during our hourly visits and appreciated having plenty of time to ask questions. The baby (we didn't know the sex) was head down for most of the late pregnancy and stayed that way—kicking vigorously as if saying "Let me out. I need more space!"

On July 2, I had mild contractions, which I assumed was false labor since the baby wasn't due for another week. These contractions continued throughout the next day, and my husband and I frantically closed down our small business. (I know! Poor planning on our part!) With the business closed at seven in the evening, the contractions came on so strong that I couldn't do anything else other than breathe. At nine in the evening, Monika pronounced me three centimeters dilated. I labored in our garden tub and in the master bedroom in bed and leaning on the walls.

Around two in the morning, I was fully dilated and started pushing. The first couple of pushes were amazing— dropping the baby multiple stations with each push. My memory gets foggy here, so I might not get this part right. At some point, my cervix was pinched between the baby's head and my body. While there are no words for this pain, Monika and Debra were calm and kept reaching into their magic bag for tools to help the labor progress. I remember feeling confident that they would figure out something to get things unstuck. One funny moment came when, after telling me to stop screaming and focus on pushing, Debra said, "Honey, I think you need to just scream it out." And I did just that. With the cervix out of the way, Monika reached for the birthing stool to help my body figure out how to push.

A little after five in the morning, I figured out pushing,

and with three big pushes, our baby slid into the world. I remember a long pause between pushes two and three when my body gathered up the strength it needed for that final push. That pause was an unexpected magical moment with our baby half-in and half-out of the world.

My baby's cord was too short to reach my breasts, so the baby hung out on my tummy while my husband and I cried and caressed her. We were so relieved that the baby had arrived that we didn't look to see the sex until Monika said, "Look! Aren't you even going to look?" But we were too busy saying hello and didn't care about much else.

Once the cord stopped pulsing and was cut, our baby girl, Cora, latched and nursed for two hours. She was pronounced a perfect ten, but proud parents that we were, we already knew that she was perfect. She looked a bit like a boxer with a squashed nose and square ears—but I'd never seen anyone so beautiful and wouldn't again until two years later when her brother was born, also at home in our bed.

Looking back, if I could tell that young momma-to-be trying to decide between multiple wonderful birth options just one thing about home birth, I would tell her this. Your pregnancy and labor will be like running a marathon—long, uncomfortable, and a mental challenge as much as a physical one. While other excellent healthcare professionals will take care of you physically, Monika will build a relationship with you that will help you prepare emotionally and mentally. And because of this relationship, when they tell you to stop screaming and push, you're going to do just that, because you trust them. While I never want to do it again, I am so thankful for the healthy home births of both of my children.

ELIZABETH'S SECOND BABY—FIRST HOME BIRTH

On Saturday, March 24, I woke up at four in the morning with contractions that were three to four minutes apart. They didn't feel strong—it actually felt like another repeat of Thursday night. I woke Ryan up to see if we should call the midwives. We waited, counted contractions, and eventually agreed to try to get more sleep and wait until they got stronger and closer together. I slept a little but was wide awake at six o'clock. The contractions, though not strong, were still three to four minutes apart. I felt excited. This had to be it! I used the bathroom and lost even more of my mucus plug and this time had bloody show (something I never experienced with my first pregnancy). I let Ryan sleep until Eleanor woke up at seven o'clock. By seven thirty, the contractions were two to three minutes apart and getting stronger. They weren't painful at all, but I had to focus through them. I alternated between leaning on my birthing ball and bouncing on it to help keep labor going. I finally felt like I was in active labor. Ryan called the midwives, alerted the birth photographer, and then called my best friend, Cassie, whom we made arrangements with to watch Eleanor while I was in labor.

Cassie arrived around eight thirty to pick up Eleanor. I gave Ella an extra hug and cried a little as she left. We told her when she came back home she'd have a little brother or sister.

Tara arrived around eight forty-five and took my vitals. Monika arrived around nine o'clock and did a vaginal exam. It was such a relief to learn that I was making good progress. I was dilated three centimeters. Contractions continued to be painless, but they were strong and came every three to four minutes. Monika was concerned that I needed rest since I hadn't slept well the night before. I lay down for a good hour and a half, listening to worship music. The midwives came in every fifteen to twenty minutes to check on baby's heart tones. Everything sounded great.

Around eleven thirty-five, Monika asked if I felt ready to get things moving. I said "Yes!" I really wanted to meet my baby. We decided to go for a walk since it was so beautiful outside. Monika, Ryan, and I walked around our block a couple times and then walked the greenbelt behind our home. It felt good to move. I'll never forget how beautiful that walk was. The bluebonnets were in bloom, the sun was shining, and I walked hand in hand with my husband through contractions. I was even able to laugh and talk in between them. I was amazed that there wasn't any pain. With Eleanor's birth, I endured excruciating back labor for hours. As we walked, I continued to focus and breathe through the contractions. They felt good. With each one, I took slow steady breaths, imagined my baby working his/her way down, and said, "I'm elastic, I'm open, this is just a muscle tightening."

Thirty minutes into our walk, I felt like we had to go home. I never stopped walking through the contractions, and I felt them beginning to strengthen and get closer together.

At 12:10 p.m., the moment we walked in the door, it was like a light switch turned on, and I immediately went into transition. I began pacing the house and moaning low moans. There still wasn't any pain, but I had to completely focus through them. Ryan called the birth photographer to let her know to come right away. Monika and Tara rushed to get the birth pool filled. I couldn't stop moving. Ryan followed me around and tried to rub my shoulders. I snapped at him to get away from me. He motioned to Tara and told her that he believed I was in second stage. At that moment, I felt the baby drop. My body was pushing the baby out by itself. I panicked and flagged down Monika. I heard her say, "Oh shit. Okay. It's time to get on the bed." The birth pool was only partially filled, so I couldn't get into it. Monika had me get on hands and knees on my bed. A few moments passed, and our birth photographer walked through the door.

While on my hands and knees, my back began to feel like it was on fire. I panicked: it felt exactly like back labor. For the first time, I felt the pain of each contraction and the baby making its way down through my pelvis. I yelled for someone to help ease the pain in my back. With Tara's help, I was able to semi-focus again and regain a little more control of the pain, which is when my water broke. It sounded like a huge water balloon exploded. I looked down to find my knees swimming in brown tinged fluid. I pushed the fear back of another hospital transfer. As Tara changed the chux pads on the bed, Monika stressed the importance of me getting off my hands and knees and birthing the baby quickly because of the meconium-stained amniotic fluid. The contractions were right on top of each other, so it felt impossible to move. Monika and Tara guided me to a side lying position, and I tried to push the baby out with the next contraction. My leg was on Ryan's shoulder and it felt all wrong. I exclaimed to Monika how horrible of a job I felt I was doing and she agreed and said I needed to be on my back. Ryan moved behind me with a pillow so I could recline on him and bring my legs up. This felt so much better! Another contraction began and after my second deep breath, I felt my body working with the contraction to push the baby down. What an amazing feeling! I almost wanted to laugh in excitement because it was completely different than my experience pushing Eleanor out. With the next contraction, the baby crowned. Monika asked me if I wanted to feel the baby's head. I said no out of fear of losing momentum. Ryan excitedly exclaimed, "The baby has a ton of hair!" With another push, the head was out, such a relief! Monika told me to push slowly with the next contraction. Both midwives helped the baby rotate as its shoulders and body were born.

Time then seemed to stop. I immediately started crying as the baby was brought to my chest. I was oblivious to the gender. All I cared about was that my baby was here. In all the commotion of cleaning up the baby and basking in the high after labor, I was shocked to hear Ryan say, "Margaret is here! We have another girl."

Less than ten minutes later, I birthed the placenta. Monika and Tara checked the placenta and cord and found that they weren't stained with meconium. Praise God! Debra, another one of my midwives, arrived a half hour later. Shortly after Debra's arrival, Ryan cut the cord. The midwives helped me get comfortable on fresh, clean sheets while Ryan got me some food. I lay with Margaret in bed for several hours, nursing and doing skin-to-skin while the midwives cleaned up and filled out the necessary paperwork. Monika examined me and found that I had a small first-degree tear to my perineum. Ryan and Candice took Margaret to the living room while I was sutured. Afterwards, Ryan and I snuggled back into bed with our sweet baby.

Margaret was born at 12:45 p.m. and was seven pounds, fourteen ounces, and twenty-one inches long. Her labor was around five hours long. I was in transition for only thirty-five minutes once we came home from our walk.

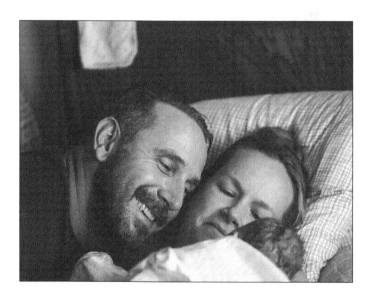

REBECCA'S FIRST BIRTH—FIRST HOME BIRTH

On the sunny August evening Laurel was born, I felt like I awoke for the first time. I cannot remember myself before, what I had done or who I was. As if I hadn't really existed until that moment. I awoke a woman within me—a fierce, determined woman who grew life, who sacrificed her own body in so many ways to bring forth another woman to grace the planet with her presence.

The hot Saturday evening before, I took a walk and observed the full moon, wondering if it was the night things would begin. Being a night owl, I went to bed after midnight, thinking I might regret the decision to stay up so late. At four thirty, I awoke to a tightening in my abdomen that came again ten minutes later, and ten minutes later. Sleep eluded me when I finally woke up my husband, Juston, at six thirty to tell him, "It's started!" He nearly jumped out of bed, asking if we should awake my mom, who had come to be with us for a few weeks. I said, "No, just keep planning on going to church." Around ten in the morning, they both said they were staying home; no way would they leave me laboring alone! By this time, the contractions were about five minutes apart.

I wandered outside for a while, walking barefoot in the lawn, sitting under the cool fan of our back patio, and enjoyed the warm sun on my face until it started becoming uncomfortable for me to sit through the contractions on my own. Juston had begun to set up the birth pool in our bedroom. I decided to call my midwife, Monika, to let her know how close together the contractions were.

She arrived a little after noon and wanted to check my progress—at three centimeters. I decided to bounce and sway on my exercise ball for a while. Time began to disappear at this point, as my focus was getting through each wave of incredible tightness. I thought I would be able to mentally get through each contraction relatively well, but the only thing helping me was saying affirmations or having my mom read them out loud to me for the duration of the wave, and having someone push on my hips/lower back. I got to a point where the only thing mentally getting me through them was simply counting—to twenty-five then to fifty—like I would climb mountains in Colorado, my motivation for getting my legs up those trails.

I sank into the warm pool for a while, leaning on the side. Monika gave me some herbal and homeopathic tinctures to help with the discomfort and help my cervix prepare. I kept telling my body to open up, open up. A little while later, she said by the sound of my contractions, she wanted to check my progress again and wondered if I wanted the rest of the birth team to come. I was uncertain if I'd need them yet; however, upon checking, I was at seven centimeters, and she said she was going to call the other midwife, June, and doula, Emily. My dear photographer friend Taylor Moss was also called to come begin documenting the journey.

I lay on the bed, on my side, to power through the intense

strength of my uterus. That incredible organ that had held, nourished, and grown my baby for forty weeks and three days was ready to finish its job. I remember Monika stepping out of the room, and Juston was with me. I felt a great contraction and my body seized like a big push. I said to Juston, "Tell Monika that was a push!" He left the room to fetch her. And here my timeline gets hazier, as I survived from one wave to the next.

Monika came back to the room and wanted to check again, and said, "Okay, we're ready to have this baby, so I'm going to have you start pushing." My heart! I was going to hold my baby soon. Taylor had arrived to take photos. Emily arrived and sat next to me on the bed, holding my hand and allowing me to crush it with each contraction. At some point, June arrived and began monitoring the baby's heartbeat with the Doppler. I labored for a while, my face tightening and throat constricted; I sat on the toilet and went through three cycles of pushing (it felt like I was going to poop the poor baby into the toilet, but there was no danger of that).

Back on the bed, striving through each wave, I would become so hot I needed a cool cloth on my forehead and neck, then the next minute I was cold. My body began to shake, so I was given sips of orange juice between contractions. Hydration was necessary, so I also drank water constantly. I hadn't wanted to labor on my back, but there I was making a magnificent effort.

Monika saw some meconium and said I needed to get the baby out; her heart rate maintained just fine. I pushed and pushed with each contraction, unearthly sounds coming out of my mouth; everyone cheered each time. This dear little head just wouldn't get past the perineum despite hot compresses and stretching with oils. I was coached to get up on my legs and squat on the bed, but even with support it was uncomfortable to me. Monika said to get on my hands and knees, and within a push, the sweet baby's head was birthed, and Monika said, "Stop pushing!" So just for a moment of inexplicable anticipation, I paused.

With the final strained push, a release came, and before me on the bed screamed my daughter, a perfectly formed human being. My immediate emotion upon seeing her lying there was shock as I thought, *there really has been a beautiful baby inside me!* I don't know what else I expected to see, but the momentary thought swiftly flew away as I picked up her vernix- and blood-smeared little body and held her to my heart; she was my heart.

It was 7:24 p.m. when Laurel Fern was born, when I awoke. This mysterious beginning of life, naturally, safe in my own home, free of medical pressure, surrounded by the people who love me and support me, and resting back in my own bed, felt so sweet and empowering. A laurel is a crown of victory; Fern was my grandma's name. This sweet, lovely babe surely is my crown of victory. I'm so grateful to have chosen a home birth with an incredible birth team. I can do anything.

MAEGAN'S FIRST BIRTH—FIRST WATER BIRTH

My water broke at six thirty on the morning of my son's due date, August 4. I remember thinking he would be born by that evening. I remember Kline started cleaning the kitchen. I called Monika, and she came over around eight o'clock and assured me I should just hang around the house, go on walks, do whatever feels right, and to start to time the contractions as they became more regular. I remember her saying it would probably be that evening.

My mom came over with tons of groceries and began to cook chicken soup. Kline went and got breakfast tacos and queso, and we snuggled on the couch, watching *Stranger Things,* and snacking most of the day.

It was beautiful and sunny and very hot that day; we went on a walk to Armadillo Park and it felt good to move. I remember the birthing coach said there would be a point in labor where a) things wouldn't be funny anymore, and b) I wouldn't want to eat anymore, and both of those things began to happen around seven in the evening.

I tried to go on another walk and could barely go down the

street before Kline held me and walked me back. It was funny how I expected my mom to be the calming force during my birth and that Kline might not know what to do, but I was totally wrong. My mom became frantic, and Kline was right by my side and made me feel so calm.

The contractions started to get closer together, and Monika came back over at eight in the evening, and I remember feeling so calm hearing her voice. I had no idea what a long night it would be. When Monika arrived, she checked my cervix, and I believe I was three centimeters dilated at that point. I remember getting in and out of the bathtub and the warm water helping the contractions ripple through my body.

The majority of the night was pretty rough and a blur, but Monika made me feel so safe and as comfortable as possible, given that I needed an IV for the strep B (or some sort of bacterial thing in my vagina canal) and that I couldn't stop throwing up. At one point, I remember being on all fours, throwing up with my IV arm in the air.

Around midnight, Monika tried to get me to rest and relax, and I took ibuprofen and a shot of whiskey and fell asleep for maybe an hour. The rest of the night is blurry. I remember getting in and out of the bathtub; I remember thinking the pain would never end.

I believe Debra arrived around five or six in the morning and had me doing squats with Kline behind me, with his arms under my armpits to support me. I remember this being one of the most bonding and pivotal moments of the birth. Kline was breathing slowly in my ear trying to get me to mimic his breathing as we squatted over and over with me in his arms. I felt like things were moving along.

I became very scared we wouldn't have the baby in time, and I would have to go to hospital. I remember Debra assuring me we were having this baby. I think around seven or eight in the morning, I began to push. Kline was lying in bed with me, holding my hand, as Monika and Debra coached me to stop pushing as the contractions ended and to breathe and not tense up.

I remember my baby's little arm got stuck and was so painful I can still feel it. We finally crowned, and Monika put my hand down to feel Walter's little head, and it felt so close! There are absolutely no words to describe what followed. The feeling of him being born was the most magical and amazing feeling of release.

They immediately put him on my chest, and it was the greatest feeling in the world. We had made it to the other side, and he was healthy and safe in our arms. Everything that came was pure magic.

I remember Debra teaching me to breastfeed and Monika checking our vitals and cleaning and getting everything organized. In no time, we were snuggled into clean sheets with the chaos of the evening completely out of sight. Monika and Debra are so professional and amazing at what they do. I felt so safe and in the right hands the whole time. Literally from the moment I met Monika, I knew I needed her.

Everything about her made me love her; she was so knowledgeable and fierce and clear, while simultaneously being patient and comforting in every way. Walter's birth was the best day of my life, and I couldn't have picked a better team of midwives to be by my side and help me through this birth of mother and son.

The days after Walter was born, Debra and Monika came and checked on us regularly, making sure he was latching and that we were both happy and healthy. I felt in such wonderful hands and when I decide to have another baby, I wouldn't have anyone else.

JESSICA'S SECOND AND THIRD BIRTH—FIRST AND SECOND HOME BIRTH

My birth story started in 2016, at thirty-two weeks pregnant. I had already met with Heart of Texas Midwives in the beginning of my pregnancy, in the hopes of having a homebirth. My family and friends persuaded me to not do so. I went along with them and chose a birthing center. By my thirty-second week, though, I had to follow my true gut and went under the care of Debra and Monika, leaving the birth center behind. They instantly made me feel very welcomed and cared for me as if I was one of their own.

At forty weeks and five days, my labor started quickly and within a couple of hours I was at seven centimeters dilated. I thought for sure I would have my baby by lunchtime. Think again! I stalled at seven centimeters for several hours. I tried my best to get my rest and sprinkle in some work to get the labor moving, such as going up and down my stairs.

We then decided to use my rebozo. Monika and Debra sifted me like a sack of flour and got me to transition very quickly! I vividly remember them both massaging my legs while I had intense contractions. I had this vision of birthing in my tub and did so on my hands and knees. As I grasped my husband's arms for pushing, my little boy was born with a few powerful pushes.

I think that the aftercare of labor is really just as important as the pre-care. I was so appreciative of them coming to my home and showing me how to tend to my child in a loving and respectful way. My first child was born in the hospital and I had zero aftercare, so this was new and refreshing. I felt supported, like I had gained two mothers and friends.

A little over a year later, I became pregnant with my third, and I immediately knew I was going to use Heart of Texas Midwives again for this third child. The focus on emotional support was so eye-opening for me. It wasn't just a clinical appointment of looking at statistics. I had a safe place to communicate my fears and stresses, which I feel is often overlooked on mothers.

With this labor, also at forty weeks and five days, I was able to do lots of outside walking and soaking in my tub, having my husband support me getting to the next stage of labor. I once again needed the help of the rebozo, due to my cervix being tilted and had a very speedy transition. The labor was so gentle; my baby was born in his amniotic sac in my own bed! I had very minimal swelling, no tearing. The aftercare was once again top of mind awareness with the midwives. It's so nice that they come to your home in your time of rest and really promote that precious postpartum period.

I could not imagine going through either of my labors in a hospital without caving in to the pressures of drugs and or epidural. Being in the comfort of your own home with your own bed, being able to move around freely to progress labor, and having the support around you in a loving and patient way is priceless.

I now have a lovely rebozo that helped with the labor of my two sons and a certain amount of trust in myself and my body that I'm strong and capable of doing it again. I'm fulfilled with my family size now, but if I could have gone back in time and had all three of my children with the midwives at home, I would.

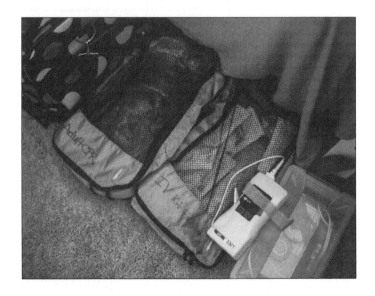

ASHLEY'S FIRST, SECOND, THIRD BIRTH—ALL HOME BIRTHS

It was one of the nicest days I remember when I birthed my first son, Colton. I woke up about five thirty in the morning with increasingly consistent labor pains and knew quickly that it was the day! I called my mom, grandma, and midwife, and my husband proceeded to get my birth tub ready.

One of my favorite memories from that day, besides seeing my baby, was walking up the street with my mom on this beautiful March day. I walked all the way up the street to my friend's house, pausing between contractions, and I remember thinking how incredibly lucky I was to be able to walk around outside on this beautiful day! The feeling of being outside and in labor was so calming and grounding, I remember feeling sad for people stuck inside a hospital and not able to experience this as I was.

It was a long-ish labor from start to finish, but it didn't feel that way, due to everything being so gradual. I got in and out of the water as my labor progressed, though I would have stayed in the whole time if I didn't need to move around to help progression!

Once I got to the more intense parts of labor, I had a shift mentally. I was now in a warrior state, so tired but pushing forward and finding a strength I didn't know I had again and again, with the guidance of my midwife who always knew just what to say to me, just how to position me so I could make it to the next stage.

There was a part when I didn't know if I could do it, if I

could move forward. It was that moment that changed my life. Being at home, being guided by a midwife, and having my family around me was the only environment in which I could have experienced the amazing strength and self-discovery that I look back to even today and gain insight from.

The last part of my labor, pushing, was a different me: focused, ready to do all I could to meet my beautiful boy. When I saw his amazing little face, I absolutely knew that my life would never be the same, not just because I had this precious new life, but because of the journey I had taken to bring him into this world and the model of care I had chosen for him and myself. I am so very thankful I chose home birth and didn't miss out on the incredible experience of natural, empowering birth.

ASHLEY'S SECOND BIRTH—SECOND HOME BIRTH

I was so excited to be in labor with my second son and to repeat this experience with my midwife. We had been through a great labor together with my first. This time, I felt more seasoned, relaxed, and confident, and I couldn't wait to "master" this birth!

I went into labor the same time as my first. Everything was relaxed and I was actually catching up on some TV shows into pretty heavy contractions, just floating in my birth tub.

Things progressed and I found myself needing to concentrate on some heavy contractions. There were some things similar, but I was struck by just how different this birth felt!

The most intense period was when my son locked his elbow, leg, something and made it difficult for him to get down the birth canal. When he finally moved, he dropped incredibly quickly, and that was very shocking to both of us! I felt a bit of panic in that moment but also knew we were very close. My midwife knew exactly how to manage this situation and was able to get the baby and me both to calm and prepare for pushing.

I am so grateful I had her expertise in that moment because without that I could see things going very differently. It was only about five minutes later that he was born. This birth really proved to me how valuable the midwife skillset really is. You never know where your birth experience will lead you, and having someone to guide you through that process who is so in tune with each phase of the birth journey is invaluable.

I always felt safe with my midwife by my side, and that allowed me to have the best possible birth experience.

On the eve of the birth of my third son, I was so sure I would have him that next day that I prepared things accordingly. I was very in tune with my body and felt like it was time! I expected that labor would start sometime that night, but early morning came and still no real contractions.

Then at seven thirty in the morning, things started to get rhythmic and it seemed like it was baby time! My other sons had a T-ball game later that morning, so I proceeded to get breakfast and get them ready, all while in early labor, while my husband got my birth tub ready and prepared for everything.

This is where things start to get comical! My husband, expecting a much longer labor, ran out to the corner store for a few items while I waited for my three-year-old to finish breakfast. The contractions were starting to get intense and I realized I was in a race against time to be able to make it back up the stairs!

So there I was, asking my soon-to-be middle child to PLEASE finish his breakfast so Mom can go upstairs and have a baby. Fortunately, we made it, and I now wanted to get in my (regular) tub right away.

This was getting to the point where I had to stop and

breathe heavily through contractions, and I needed water relief! I was in the tub, my kids were running around gathering their baseball items, my husband was back; things were chaotic but evening out.

Just a few minutes in the water and I was starting to feel very intense, low contractions, and I suddenly felt trapped in that tub and needed to get out NOW.

Naturally, at that moment, my then youngest decided to jump on our bed and hit his head. I was drying off, soothing a crying child, tucking in a baseball uniform, and breathing through contractions that I could barely stand through!

Meanwhile, my husband was frantically filling up the birth tub because it was apparent this baby wasn't waiting. I finally got some clothes on and leaned next to the bed in very heavy labor.

My midwife walked in at that moment and I don't think I've ever been happier to see anyone! I was a little frazzled from the chaos and incredibly quick progression of labor, and I remember her whispering to me, "I'm here. You're safe. You're safe."

Everything immediately slowed and I was able to get in my "birth zone" very quickly. It was amazing the way she was able to focus my energy, and that gave me the power to cope with my very fast labor.

It wasn't long before I was pushing, and just a few minutes later my sweet new boy was born. (We didn't get my birth tub filled in time, but it worked out just fine!)

It was a great birth experience and I actually love the chaos and comedy that surround his story. That's real life! The ease in which he was brought into the world is a great testament to midwives and home birth. It was natural and beautiful and made possible by the intuitions and expertise of a great midwife who knows what to do no matter what she's walking into!

Conclusion

Now that you have journeyed with me into my world of home birth, you know that you have a choice about where to birth your baby.

On our journey through this book, you have learned that home birth is safe when you hire a licensed and skilled midwife. Statistics confirm that home birth is safe.

Prenatal care with a midwife is comprehensive and thorough. The pillars of midwifery-led care are built on relationship, nutrition, exercise, mental health, and midwife as a facilitator and educator. The continuous continuity of care allows midwives to give individualized care based on the woman and her family's needs.

Women who birth at home commit to the sensations of birth and work in unison with their bodies to birth their babies. The comfort of their home, the freedom of movement, loving support, and staying hydrated and nourished allows them to do the work. The midwives monitor the well-being of mom and baby during the home birth process. Midwives are the guardians of normal pregnancy and childbirth, recognize variations of normal, redirect to bring back to the range of normal, or transfer to the medical community when the need arises.

You learned about the best-kept secret of all—postpartum care at home. Postpartum care at home with a midwife is thorough and allows you to bond and rest with your baby. Most of all, it gives you a great chance at a successful breastfeeding relationship with your baby.

During our journey, you met Amy and Lisa, who had babies under the medical model of care and midwifery model of care. Both women were happy with their experiences and the choices they made.

Toward the end of the book, you met some of the wonderful people I served as a home birth midwife.

My desire in writing this book is that you now understand home birth better and regard it as a safe option to birth a baby.

Whether you are considering a home birth or know someone who is planning a home birth, you can feel good about home birth in knowing this is a safe choice. Your next step is to meet a home birth midwife.

Please share this book! It is time to open the door wide to the choice of home birth for women and their families.

We cannot choose what we do not know.

We cannot judge what we do not understand.

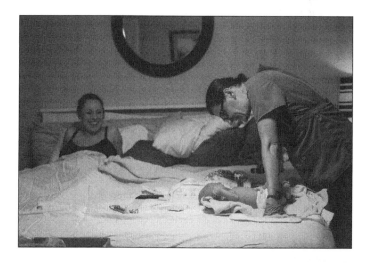

Acknowledgments

Thank you to all the women and families who choose home birth.

Thank you to all clients past, present, and future, who invite me to go on a journey with them.

Thank you to all home birth midwives past, present, and future; we are united in love for women, babies, and families. We are bonded in our passion for holding the space and therefore never truly alone in the dead of night when we lie awake, watching and waiting while the world sleeps.

Thank you to Veronica and Tucker for believing in this book and encouraging me to move forward with the impossible dream.

Thank you to Scribe and its editors, who led the way for me.

Thank you to Kristen for being the best companion on this journey anyone could ever dream of.

Thank you to Mary for believing in me and being the greatest mentor I could ever have.

Thank you to Marti and Dave for the courage to believe in home birth.

Thank you to the doctors who accept our home birth transfers in Austin, Texas, for leading the way to safe home births.

Thank you to St. David's hospitals and their nurses in Austin, Texas, for accepting home birth transfers and making home birth safer.

Thank you to my midwife partners, June, Lynne, and Debra, for their support and willingness to journey with mommies and babies who choose home birth.

Thank you to my parents, whose courage and drive continue to inspire me.

Thank you, last but not least, to my brother, Sepp, the best brother any sister could ever have. You have always believed in me and for that I will always be grateful.

Resources

"Recent Declines in Induction of Labor by Gestational Age," Data table for Figure 1. Induction of labor, by gestational age: United States, 1990–2012. *NCHS Data Brief*, Number 155.

American College of Nurse Midwives. www.midwife.org.

American College of Nurse-Midwives. "Comparison of Certified Nurse-Midwives, Certified Midwives, Certified Professional Midwives Clarifying the Distinctions Among Professional Midwifery Credentials in the U.S." http://www.midwife.org/acnm/files/ccLibraryFiles/FILENAME/000000006807/FINAL-ComparisonChart-Oct2017.pdf.

American College of Nurse-Midwives. "Definition of Midwifery and Scope of Practice of Certified Nurse-Midwives and Certified Midwives." http://www.midwife.org/ACNM/files/ACNMLibraryData/UPLOADFILENAME/000000000266/Definition of Midwifery and Scope of Practice of CNMs and CMs Dec 2011.pdf

American College of Nurse-Midwives. "Fact Sheet CNM/CM-attended Birth Statistics in the United States." http://www.midwife.org/acnm/files/ccLibraryFiles/Filename/000000005950/CNM-CM-AttendedBirths-2014-031416FINAL.pdf.

American College of Nurse-Midwives. Provision of Home Birth
Services, *Clinical Bulletin* 61 (November 2015).

Bonaparte, Alicia D. "The Persecution and Prosecution of Granny
Midwives In South Carolina, 1900–1940." Dissertation. https://
etd.library.vanderbilt.edu/available/etd-07252007-122217/
unrestricted/bonapartedissertation2007final.pdf

Centers for Disease Control and Prevention. "Causes of
Infant Mortality." August 3, 2018. https://www.cdc.gov/
reproductivehealth/maternalinfanthealth/infantmortality.
htm#causes.

Centers for Disease Control and Prevention. "CDC Activities."
August 3, 2018. https://www.cdc.gov/reproductivehealth/
maternalinfanthealth/infantmortality.htm#cdc

Centers for Disease Control and Prevention. "Grief Resources."
August 3, 2018. https://www.cdc.gov/reproductivehealth/
maternalinfanthealth/infantmortality.htm#grief.

Centers for Disease Control and Prevention. "Infant Mortality
Rates by State, 2016." https://www.cdc.gov/reproductivehealth/
maternalinfanthealth/infantmortality.htm#rates

Centers for Disease Control and Prevention. "Infant Mortality
Rates by Race and Ethnicity, 2016." August 3, 2018. https://
www.cdc.gov/reproductivehealth/maternalinfanthealth/
infantmortality.htm#chart.

Centers for Disease Control and Prevention. "Infant Mortality."
August 3, 2018. https://www.cdc.gov/reproductivehealth/
maternalinfanthealth/infantmortality.htm#about.

Citizens for Midwifery. "New Home Birth Study from the MANA
Statistics Dataset Shows That Planned Home Birth with Skilled
Midwives is Safe for Low-Risk Pregnancies." 2014. http://www.
cfmidwifery.org/pdf/MANAHBData04-09FactSheet.pdf.

Hamilton, Brady E., Joyce A. Martin, and Michelle J.K. Osterman. "Births: Preliminary Data for 2015." *National Vital Statistics Reports* 65, no. 3 (2016): 1-15.

MacDorman, Marian F., T.J. Mathews, and Eugene Declercq. "Trends in Out-of-Hospital Births in the United States, 1990–2012." *NCHS Data Brief* 144 (2014): 1-8.

Martin, Joyce A., Hamilton, Brady E., Osterman, Michelle J.K., Driscoll, Anne K., and T.J. Matthews. "Births: Final Data for 2015." *National Vital Statistics Reports, (NVSS)*, 66, no. 1, January 5, 2017.

Midwives Alliance North America. "Standards and Qualifications for the Art and Practice of Midwifery," October 2, 2005. https://mana.org/pdfs/MANAStandardsQualificationsColor.pdf.

Midwives Alliance North America. www.mana.org.

North American Registry of Midwives. www.narm.org.

NPR. "Focus On Infants During Childbirth Leaves U.S. Moms In Danger." *Lost Mothers: Maternal Mortality in the U.S.* https://www.npr.org/2017/05/12/527806002/focus-on-infants-during-childbirth-leaves-u-s-moms-in-danger.

Osterman, Michelle J.K. and Joyce A. Martin. "Epidural and Spinal Anesthesia Use During Labor:27-state Reporting Area, 2008." *National Vital Statistics Reports (NVSS)*, 59, no. 5, April 6, 2011.

Rubinstein, Nechama. "Midwifery Provision of Home Birth Services: The Untold Story of the Hebrew Midwives and the Exodus - Biblical Women." *Chabad.org*, https://www.chabad.org/theJewishWoman/article_cdo/aid/1465248/jewish/The-Untold-Story-of-the-Hebrew-Midwives-and-the-Exodus.htm

Texas Department of Licensing and Regulation. "Midwives." https://www.tdlr.texas.gov/midwives/midwives.htm

The American College of Obstetrics and Gynecologists. "Committee Opinion on Planned Home Birth." No. 697, April 2017.

The Big Push for Midwives Campaign. "CPMS Legal Status by State." June 2017. http://PushForMidwives.org

The Midwives Alliance Core Competencies, revised 2014, https://mana.org/pdfs/MANACoreCompetenciesFINAL.pdf.

About the Author

MONIKA STONE, CPM, LM is a home birth midwife in Austin, Texas, where she resides with her husband of nineteen years and her two children, born at home. She is licensed through the Texas Department of Licensing and Regulation (TDLR) and the North American Registry of Midwives (NARM). She was born and raised outside Munich, Germany where she was trained as a pediatric nurse in Munich, Germany. Monika worked as a Birth Doula in Austin for eight years before she became a midwife. She was trained through the Association of Texas Midwives Training Program, where she graduated as Student of the Year in 2011. She has been the primary midwife to hundreds of women and has caught hundreds of babies at home.

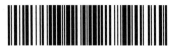